Molecular Bases of Neurodegenerative Disorders of the Retina

Edited by:

Hemant Khanna, Ph.D.

Department of Ophthalmology, University of Massachusetts
Medical School, Worcester, MA 01605, USA

General:

1. Any dispute or claim arising out of or in connection with this License Agreement or the Work (including non-contractual disputes or claims) will be governed by and construed in accordance with the laws of the U.A.E. as applied in the Emirate of Dubai. Each party agrees that the courts of the Emirate of Dubai shall have exclusive jurisdiction to settle any dispute or claim arising out of or in connection with this License Agreement or the Work (including non-contractual disputes or claims).
2. Your rights under this License Agreement will automatically terminate without notice and without the need for a court order if at any point you breach any terms of this License Agreement. In no event will any delay or failure by Bentham Science Publishers in enforcing your compliance with this License Agreement constitute a waiver of any of its rights.
3. You acknowledge that you have read this License Agreement, and agree to be bound by its terms and conditions. To the extent that any other terms and conditions presented on any website of Bentham Science Publishers conflict with, or are inconsistent with, the terms and conditions set out in this License Agreement, you acknowledge that the terms and conditions set out in this License Agreement shall prevail.

Bentham Science Publishers Ltd.
Executive Suite Y - 2
PO Box 7917, Saif Zone
Sharjah, U.A.E.
Email: subscriptions@benthamscience.org

BENTHAM SCIENCE

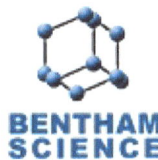

CONTENTS

PREFACE

The interpretation of light signals has fascinated as well as perplexed the minds of geniuses, including Isaac Newton, Albert Einstein and Charles Darwin. The eye is the medium through which our brain interprets the various environmental cues. It also acts as a window to the brain. Ever since humanity has developed an understanding of the ways eyes interpret light signals, many mysteries about its structure, development and function have been unearthed.

Photoreceptors (rods and cones) - which are situated in the back of the eye in a transparent tissue called Retina - form the majority of the neurons that are involved in transmitting light signals to the brain. The unique polarized morphology and physiology of the photoreceptors make them one of the most fascinating cell types. So much so, that they have been used to examine the way our eyes have evolved to interpret visual cues. In fact, photoreceptors are the first responders to light, and thus hold the bulk of our visual power. However, 'with great power comes great responsibility'; photoreceptors have evolved stringent mechanisms to maintain their function over the lifespan of an organism. The light-sensing cellular antenna of the photoreceptors is a modified cilium. Even slight perturbations in the development, structure, or function of the cilium can result in severe blindness disorders (called ciliopathies). Innovative technological advances are rapidly leading to a better understanding of the photoreceptors, particularly with respect to the involvement of the cilia in interpreting the light signal. Moreover, defects in the retinal vasculature and neuronal degeneration are the primary cause of debilitating disorders, such as Diabetic Retinopathy and Age-related Macular Degeneration. Numerous investigations have yielded new insights on the involvement of defective protein trafficking and angiogenesis in the manifestation of various eye diseases. I have compiled information from excellent investigators who have worked diligently and made seminal contributions to the field of photoreceptor development and pathogenesis of neuronal degeneration in the retina.

My sincere thanks go to the authors for contributing chapters and highlighting their comprehensive and cutting-edge research.

Cover art by Manisha Anand, Department of Ophthalmology, UMASS Medical School, Worcester, MA.

Hemant Khanna
Department of Ophthalmology,
UMASS Medical School,
Worcester, MA,
USA

List of Contributors

Brian D. Perkins	Department of Ophthalmic Research, Cole Eye Institute, Cleveland Clinic 9500 Euclid Ave, Cleveland, OH, USA
Cathleen Wallmuth	Indiana University School of Medicine, 1160 W. Michigan St, Indianapolis, IN, USA
Hemant Khanna	Department of Ophthalmology, University of Massachusetts Medical School, Worcester, MA, USA
Hongwei Ma	Department of Cell Biology, University of Oklahoma Health Sciences Center, Oklahoma City, OK, USA
Inderjeet Kaur	Brien Holden Eye Research Centre, LV Prasad Eye Institute Hyderabad, India
Jeanne M. Frederick	Department of Ophthalmology and Visual Sciences, University of Utah Health Science Center, Salt Lake City, UT 84132, USA
Jay K Chhablani	Smt Kannuri Santhamma Centre for Vitreo Retinal diseases, LV Prasad Eye Institute Hyderabad, India
Li Jiang	Department of Ophthalmology and Visual Sciences, University of Utah Health Science Center, Salt Lake City, UT 84132, USA
Martin Biel	Center for Integrated Protein Science Munich (CIPSM), Department of Pharmacy-Center for Drug Research Ludwig-Maximilians-Universität München Munich, Germany
Michael W. Stuck	Department of Cell Biology, University of Oklahoma Health Sciences Center, Oklahoma City, OK, USA
Muna I. Naash	University of Houston, Department of Biomedical Engineering 3517 Cullen Blvd. Room 2027, Houston, TX, USA
Na Luo	Indiana University School of Medicine, 1160 W. Michigan St., Indianapolis, IN, USA
Raju V.S. Rajala	Departments of Ophthalmology Physiology, and Cell Biology, University of Oklahoma Health Sciences Center and Dean A. McGee Eye Institute, Oklahoma City, OK, USA
Shahna Shahulhameed	Brien Holden Eye Research Centre, LV Prasad Eye Institute Hyderabad, India
Shannon M. Conley	Department of Cell Biology, University of Oklahoma Health Sciences Center, Oklahoma City, OK, USA
Stylianos Michalakis	Center for Integrated Protein Science Munich (CIPSM), Department of Pharmacy-Center for Drug Research Ludwig-Maximilians-Universität München, Munich, Germany
Subhabrata Chakrabarti	Brien Holden Eye Research Centre, LV Prasad Eye Institute Hyderabad, India
Wolfgang Baehr	Department of Ophthalmology and Visual Sciences, University of Utah Health Science Center, Salt Lake City, UT, USA
Xi-Qin Ding	Department of Cell Biology, University of Oklahoma Health Sciences Center, Oklahoma City, OK, USA
Yang Sun	Indiana University School of Medicine, 1160 W. Michigan St., Indianapolis, IN, USA

CHAPTER 1

Ciliary Trafficking in Vertebrate Photoreceptors

Hemant Khanna[*]

Department of Ophthalmology, UMASS Medical School, Worcester, MA, USA

Abstract: Cilia are microtubule-based extensions of the plasma membrane of cells. These extensions detect extrinsic cues that are crucial for carrying out a myriad of developmental and homeostatic signaling cascades. Cilia have evolved diverse means to mediate signaling cascades in a cell-type specific manner. In this article, I have summarized the conserved mechanisms of formation of cilia and their structural and functional specialization for light detection.

Keywords: Basal body, Cilia, Photoreceptor, Retina.

INTRODUCTION

The cilia, Latin for 'eyelash', were first described by Anton van Leeuwenhoek in 1675 as *'incredibly thin feet, or little legs, which were moved very nimbly'* [1]. Historically, although cilia were considered vestigial, notable hypotheses were put forth to understand the nature and function of cilia. For example, cilia were thought to be active organelles and that sperm flagella (or cilia) contained fibrils that extended across the entire length of the flagellum. However, these hypotheses could not be tested due to the technical limitations at the time. Cilia and flagella have now been recognized as key players in organism development and homeostasis [2].

Based on the structure and function of the microtubule skeleton, there are two types of cilia: motile cilia and primary (or immotile) cilia. As the name implies, motile cilia are involved in cell movement, such as sperm motility and mucosal clearance by the trachea. They originate from the basal body, the mother centriole in the form of microtubule extensions. The motile cilia possess 9 outer doublet microtubules and a central pair of singlet microtubules, forming a 9+2 array. Unlike motile cilia, the primary cilia display a 9+0 arrangement of microtubules due to the absence of the central microtubule pair. Both types of cilia are involved

[*] **Corresponding author Hemant Khanna:** Department of Ophthalmology, Albert Sherman Center AS6-2043, 368 Plantation St, Worcester, MA 01605, USA; Tel: (508)　856-8991; Fax: (508) 856-1552; E-mail: hemant.khanna@umassmed.edu

in sensory perception, hence also termed sensory cilia. Although the motile and primary cilia are clearly distinguished based upon their motility and function, there are instances of motile cilia being sensory, such as tracheal cilia, and primary cilia show properties of motility, such as the cilia in the embryonic node [3 - 7].

Cilia act as a hub for G-protein coupled receptors (GPCRs) such as rhodopsin [8 - 10]. A conserved process called Intraflagellar Transport (IFT) regulates cilia growth and function. IFT in cilia participates in signaling pathways by concentrating cognate receptor proteins in the ciliary membrane [6] and involves movement of cargo (membrane receptors) towards cilia tip by anterograde motor Kinesin-II and back to the base driven by cytoplasmic dynein-2 motor. Previous studies have shown that IFT proteins are organized into two distinct complexes: complex A (IFT144, 140, 139, and 122) and complex B (comprising of several IFT proteins, including IFT88, 81, 80, 27, and 20) [11 - 14] (Fig. **1**). Disruption of IFT proteins results in defective cilia formation and associated function.

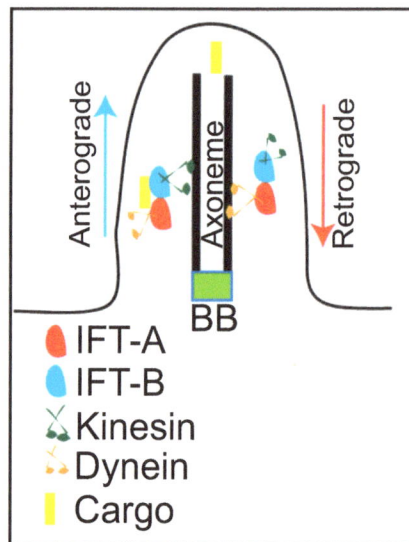

Fig. (1). Cilia: This figure depicts a simplified representation of IFT in cilia. The IFT-B particle carries cargo in anterograde direction to distal tip of cilia using the anterograde motor Kinesin-II whereas dynein and the IFT-A complex carry out retrograde movement.

Given the involvement of cilia in various developmental pathways, their dysfunction is associated with severe human disorders, collectively termed ciliopathies. In fact, involvement of cilia in human diseases was first reported in a disorder of ciliary motility in patients with primary cilia dyskinesia (PCD). Although named as a dysfunction of primary cilia, which are immotile cilia, this disease is caused due to defects in motile cilia [15]. Bjorn Afzelius first identified this disorder in 1976 in patients that exhibited immotility of bronchial cilia, sperm dysfunction and ear infections [16]. PCD in association with *situs inversus* (reversal of the left-right asymmetry of the body) is also observed in patients with Kartagener syndrome [16 - 18]. In the last decade, ciliary dysfunction has been linked to numerous ciliopathies, including Meckel-Gruber syndrome, Bardet-Biedl Syndrome, Joubert Syndrome, polycystic kidney diseases, Nephrono-phthisis, Senior-Loken Syndrome, Usher Syndrome, and some forms of Retinitis Pigmentosa (RP) [3].

RP is a clinically and genetically heterogeneous group of disorders characterized by retinal degeneration due to the loss of rod and cone photoreceptors. Photoreceptor dysfunction and degeneration due to ciliary dysfunction is commonly observed in ciliopathies. In this chapter, I will briefly describe the anatomy of the eye and the retina, and focus on the involvement of cilia in the maintenance of photoreceptor structure and function. I will also briefly discuss the involvement of ciliary function in other cell types of the retina that are critical for normal vision.

Eye

The eyeball is located at a strategic position to ensure maximum light detection while securely positioned in the cavity of the orbit. It is largely divided into anterior and posterior chambers. Light enters the anterior part of the eye, which includes the cornea and the pupil, and passes through the lens to the posterior part of the eye, which is the retina; here, it activates a complex set of events. The retina then projects the signal *via* the optic nerve to the lateral geniculate nucleus (LGN) in the brain (Fig. **2**).

There are three major fluid-filled chambers in the eye: anterior chamber, which is between the cornea and the iris; posterior chamber, between the iris and the lens and vitreous chamber, which is located between the lens and the retina and is filled with vitreous humor. The anterior and the posterior chambers are filled with a fluid called aqueous humor, which supplies nutrients to the cornea and the lens and maintains optimum pressure in the eye, called intraocular pressure (IOP). The IOP is regulated by a balanced inflow and outflow of aqueous humor from the anterior chamber into the blood stream. A major pathway for outflow of the fluid is *via* the trabecular meshwork tissue into Schlemm's canal. This outflow is measured to calculate the IOP of the eye, which serves as an important risk factor for developing an incurable blindness disorder called glaucoma [19, 20].

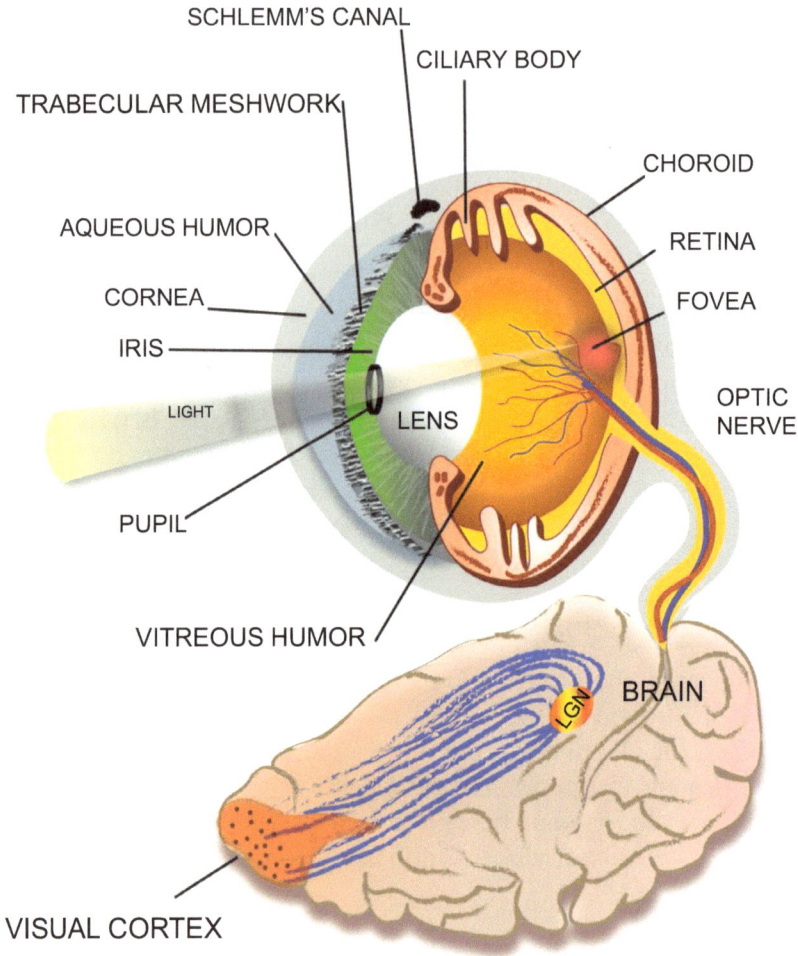

Fig. (2). Structure of the eye. The anterior and posterior parts of the eye are represented here. The optic nerve in the back of the eye traverses to the LGN in the brain to transmit the signals to the visual cortex.

Retina

The retina is the light-sensitive tissue situated in the back of the eye. It is composed of five major layers, encompassing the photoreceptor cell bodies (outer nuclear layer), the inter neurons (inner nuclear layer, consisting of both excitatory and inhibitory neurons, such as bipolar cells, amacrine cells, and horizontal cells), and the retinal ganglion cells (Fig. **3**). The neural connections with dendrites and axons of the neurons are interspersed in the outer and inner plexiform layers. The light signal is processed by the photoreceptors and the change in membrane potential is relayed to the bipolar cells and then to the ganglion cells. Along the way, lateral interactions are mediated by horizontal and amacrine cells, which provide spatial cues and lateral inhibition for correct image formation.

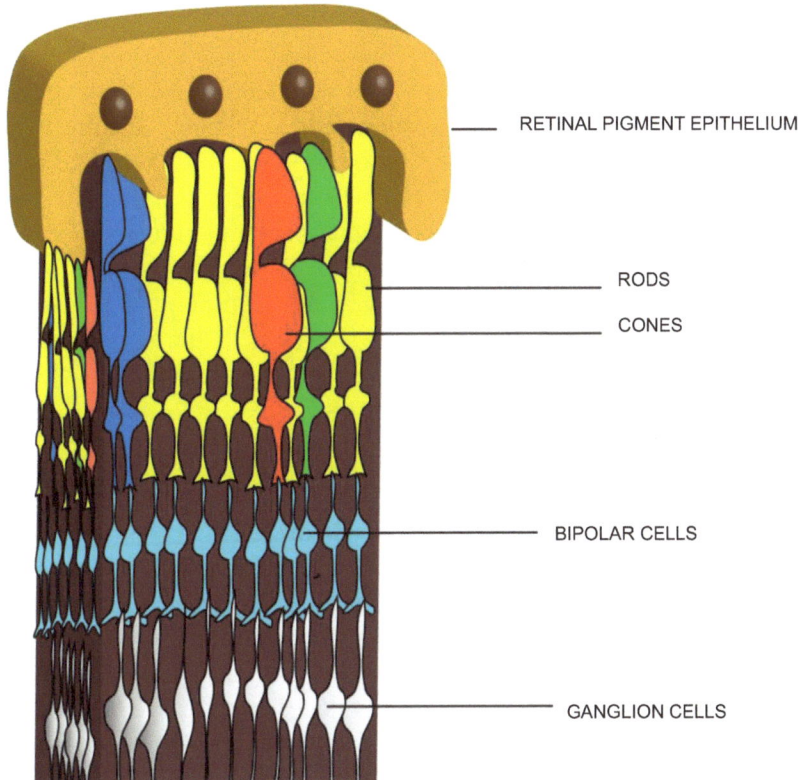

Fig. (3). Cross section of the retina: The retina is composed of various layers of neurons as indicated. Overlaying the neurons is the retinal pigment epithelium, which supplies nourishment to the photoreceptors (rods and cones). The Ganglion cells extend the optic nerve to the brain.

Photoreceptors

Photoreceptors are the most abundant cell types in the retina. There are two types of photoreceptors: rods and cones. Rods are involved in starlight or dim light vision whereas cones assist in high acuity daytime vision. The photopigment rhodopsin is expressed specifically by rods and is the most abundant protein in these neurons. The human retina contains about 120 million rods and approximately 6 million cones [21]. Depending upon the species, there are different cone subtypes, which express photopigments (opsins) that respond to specific wavelengths of light. For example, Short wave length (S; blue)-opsin expressing S-cones, Medium wave length (M; green)-opsin expressing M cones and Long wave length (L; red)-opsin expressing L cones. Primates have all three kinds of cones whereas mice only have S- and M-cones. Sequence analysis of these photopigments has revealed considerable homology and identity among the cone opsins as well as between cone opsins and rhodopsin. In fact, the L and M cone opsins share 96% identity in their amino acid sequence, indicating that they were likely derived from a gene duplication event about 30 million years ago [22 - 24].

Although we spend the majority of our life in well-lit environment in which only cones are functional, the human retina has a dearth of cones as compared to rods. Evolution has taken care of this skewed ratio by developing a central region in the retina, called the macula (and the central 2-3 millimeters called the fovea). This region contains only cones and no rods. Outside the macula, rods outnumber the cones. Additionally, the fovea lacks S-cones, which form ~10% of the cone population. These adaptations have led to the development of a strong and high acuity central vision due to the cones and a blurry peripheral vision mediated by the rods [25]. Rods play crucial roles in the maintenance of cone health and cone death induced retinal remodeling [26 - 29].

Vertebrate Photoreceptors: Modified Ciliary Neurons

Vertebrate photoreceptors are highly polarized neurons with distinct compartments for protein and lipid synthesis and for light detection. Morphologically, the photoreceptors can be divided into three major compartments: outer segment (OS), inner segment (IS), and the synaptic compartment. The bulk of protein synthesis and respiratory machinery is in the IS of the photoreceptors. All proteins and lipids necessary for the OS or the synaptic function are synthesized in the IS and then vectorially transported to their destinations. Components necessary for light detection are in the OS of the photoreceptors.

The OS is also considered a modified sensory cilium. This is because the OS shares a conserved relationship, both morphologically and physiologically, to other sensory cilia. OS formation begins when the basal body (consisting of triplet microtubules) docks at the apical region of the IS. The photoreceptor membrane forms a thin tongue-shaped microvillus extensions of the apical portion of the inner segment, which resemble the calyx of a flower. Hence, these structures are named calycal processes [30]. On the lateral walls of the ridge of the inner segment plasma membrane from which the cilium grows there are highly ordered structures forming a periciliary ridge complex (PRC). These ridges were later found to contain large molecular weight protein complexes, such as the usherin complexes [31 - 33].

Photoreceptors exhibit a unique property of accumulation of numerous filament, tubule and vesicle-like structures in the distal cilium. These structures successively transform into sac-like structures, called rod sacs, which then form the flattened array of membranous discs. Another intriguing early observation was the asymmetrical nature of the early stages of OS development. It was found that rod sacs, which later form the mature OS discs, develop on one side of the cilium while the other side remains largely undifferentiated [34]. Molecular mechanisms underlying such asymmetry in ciliary extension remain elusive to date. A distinguishing feature between a rod and a cone OS is that the rod discs are largely closed and are inside the ciliary membrane whereas ultrastructural analysis of the cone OS identified orderly stack of membranous lamellae that are continuous with the ciliary membrane. Some studies however, have revealed closed cone OS discs [35, 36]. Other than the morphological differences, the cytoskeletal arrangement seems similar between a rod and a cone OS.

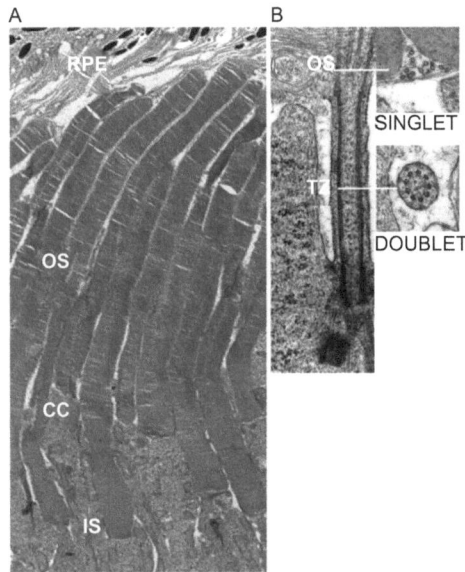

Fig. (4). Ultrastructure of the photoreceptors. Transmission electron microscopy of adult mouse photoreceptors shows a densely-packed array of discs in the outer segment (OS) in A. Panel B depicts a transition zone (TZ) and OS of a photoreceptor. Insets show the cross sections from the TZ (doublet microtubule array) and the base of the OS (singlet microtubules). RPE: retinal pigment epithelium; IS: inner segment.

Elegant studies have revealed the protein and lipid composition of the discs [37 - 46]. Given that photoreceptors are postmitotic neurons and are constantly processing light signal, they are under immense oxidative. It has been postulated that photoreceptors have evolved a mechanism of shedding of their distal tips and subsequent phagocytosis by the RPE (retinal pigment epithelium) to reduce the stress. To compensate for this loss of OS membranes, new discs are synthesized at the base of the OS, which requires additional protein and lipid generation and directional trafficking to the OS. Work by Richard Young, Dean Bok and colleagues revealed that the periodic shedding of the distal 10% of the OS tips in mice and phagocytosis by the RPE in conjunction with the subsequent renewal proximally confers long-term survival and maintenance of photoreceptor function. Similar processes are believed to occur in cone OS as well [47 - 49]. However, molecular mechanisms underlying disc formation are not completely understood. This is largely because photoreceptors are the only cell types that exhibit such a phenomenon and thus, it is hard to recapitulate such conditions *in vitro*. Moreover, structural constraints and tissue processing procedures make it difficult to carefully assess the mechanisms of disc formation and arrangement in intact OS.

Nonetheless, the first model to explain this complex phenomenon was proposed by Steinberg *et al.* (1980) [50], which was later supported with some evidence by Matsumoto and Besharse (1985) [51]. This model, termed 'evagination model' proposed that new discs are formed by evagination of the basal OS plasma membrane based on the observation of open discs during ultrastructural analyses. After about 22 years, Ching-Hwa Sung and colleagues proposed an alternative model called 'vesicular targeting model', according to which rhodopsin-containing vesicles associated with Smad Anchor for receptor Activation (SARA), syntaxin 3 and phosphatidylinositol 3-phosphate (PI3P) are incorporated into discs during disc formation. This model posits an absence of open nascent discs and that disc formation and rhodopsin incorporation occur simultaneously inside the OS [52, 53]. Although vesicles at the base of the OS were not observed in a subsequent cryo-electron tomography analysis of 3D maps of mammalian photoreceptor cilium, absence of 'open discs' was confirmed in that analysis [54]. A series of recent publications have further examined the mode of disc morphogenesis in vertebrate species. These studies provide compelling evidence for the evagination model for disc morphogenesis in rod photoreceptors [55 - 57].

Phototransduction: A Ciliary Phenomenon

The opsin molecule, a G protein coupled receptor, is inserted in the disc membrane and dos not respond to light until bound to the light-sensitive chromophore 11-*cis* retinal. Photon capture by the chromophore causes it to isomerize to all-*trans* retinal, resulting in a conformational change in the opsin (Metarhodopsin II). This step is the only light-dependent step in the cascade. Metarhodopsin II dissociates from the retinal and diffuses in the disc membrane where it interacts with the GDP-bound small GTPase transducin. This interaction activates transducin to bind to GTP, which subsequently dissociate into GTP-bound α-subunit (Tα-GTP) and a $\beta\gamma$ subunit (T$\beta\gamma$). Tα-GTP associates with cyclic nucleotide phosphodiesterase, which leads to the hydrolysis of cGMP. In the dark, the concentration of cGMP, which serves as a messenger to the plasma membrane, is high, which results in an influx of Na^+ and Ca^{2+} ions through the depolarized open cyclic nucleotide gated channel. However, the decrease in the cGMP concentration due to its hydrolysis in light results in the closure of the CNG channel, consequent decrease in the Na^+ and Ca^{2+} concentration and hyperpolarization of the cell. This leads to the decrease in the release of the neurotransmitter, thereby initiating the neural signal. Additional mechanisms are also in place to terminate the cascade. The signal is transmitted by synaptic activity to the inner neurons: bipolar cells, amacrine cells, horizontal cells and in the end to output neurons called retinal ganglion cells. The axons of the ganglion cells transmit the information to the brain by forming the optic nerve [20, 21, 58, 59].

In addition to the phototransduction cascade, the photoreceptor cilia also communicate with the RPE to regenerate the chromophore. The all-*trans* retinol dissociated from Metarhodopsin-II is transported to the RPE, where it goes through a series of well-described reactions, mediated by enzymes such as RPE65 and LRAT to 11-*cis* retinol and subsequently to 11-*cis* retinal, which is subsequently transported back to the OS. This portion of the signaling cascade is called visual cycle [19].

Cilia in Other Cell Types Involved in Vision

As detailed above, massive amount of work has been done to understand the role of cilia in photoreceptor biology. This is largely because of the overwhelming majority of photoreceptors in the retina. In a recent study, presence of primary cilia in other mouse retinal cell types was investigated using specific antibodies against marker proteins. Ciliary staining was observed, in addition to photoreceptors, in the synaptic layer and ganglion cell layer [60]. These invest-igations also suggest that the synapses may share features of cilia and the inner retinal cell types may not necessarily develop cilia as organelles. Interestingly, primary cilia were detected in rat Muller glia and defects in ciliary function was shown to affect the proliferation and dedifferentiation of these cell types in culture [61]. Additional investigations are necessary to unravel the presence and function of cilia in other retinal cell types.

Retinal Pigment Epithelium (RPE)

RPE cells in culture are shown to form primary cilia. In fact, cultured RPE cells are used as a model to examine cilia biogenesis and function [62]. However, the *in vivo* role of cilia in the RPE is not completely understood. In fact, the localization of cilia in the RPE is technically challenging due to the formation of apical processes in the apical RPE. If cilia are also present, they might be involved in sensing the signals from the OS tips during phagocytosis. One study showed that rat RPE develops cilia transiently during rat development and this ciliogenesis is associated with expression levels of the Claudin protein [63]. Hence, it is possible that cilia perform a developmental role in RPE-retina interaction.

Endothelial Cells

The retina is separated from blood vessels by the blood-retinal barrier. This is divided into two parts: inner barrier, which is composed of the retinal capillary endothelial cells, Muller glia and the pericytes and nourishes the inner retina, and outer barrier, which is formed by the RPE cells between outer retina and the choroidal endothelial blood vessels [64]. Disruption of the blood retinal barrier is associated with devastating blindness diseases, diabetic retinopathy and neo-vascular AMD (age-related macular degeneration). In DR, the damage to the blood vessels of the retina occurs due to diabetic complications. On the other hand, AMD is a slow and progressive loss of vision that usually starts in old age (~60 years or older). The vision problems happen due to the loss of the photoreceptors in the macular (central) region of the retina. One mechanism of DR and AMD progression is angiogenesis, which is the expansion of existing blood vessels, from retinal or choroidal endothelial cells. It has been shown that endothelial cells form primary cilia, which act as shear stress sensors in response to blood flow [65]. It would be interesting to assess any possible relationship between endothelial cilia and the pathogenesis of DR and AMD has not been examined.

Anterior Segment

A recent study from Young Sun and colleagues demonstrated the involvement of cilia and ciliary signaling in the maintenance of intraocular pressure (IOP), aberrations in which are associated with the pathogenesis of glaucoma [66]. It was found that trabecular meshwork cells in the anterior segment of the eye, which regulates intraocular pressure by draining the majority of aqueous fluid, form primary cilia and that mechanosensation by these cilia is involved in regulating the IOP. In addition to the trabecular meshwork, primary cilia are also found in the corneal endothelium and are believed to be involved in maintaining corneal function [67].

CONCLUDING REMARKS

The photoreceptors develop a specialized sensory cilium in the form of light-sensing outer segments. These cilia are unique both in terms of morphology as well as structural and functional maintenance. Defects in the generation or maintenance of photoreceptor cilia result in severe blindness disorders.

Knowledge of the mechanisms by which the photoreceptor cilia adopt such unique characteristics will provide clues to not only understand the fundamental mechanisms of cilia function but will also assist in designing therapeutic intermediates for the diverse ciliopathies.

LIST OF ABBREVIATIONS

OS   outer segment

IS   inner segment

ONL   outer nuclear layer

LGN   lateral geniculate nucleate

DR   diabetic retinopathy

AMD   age-related macular degeneration

IOP   intraocular pressure

TZ   transition zone

CC   connecting cilium

CONFLICT OF INTEREST

The author (editor) declares no conflict of interest, financial or otherwise.

ACKNOWLEDGEMENTS

This study is supported by grants from the National Institutes of Health (EY022372) and Foundation Fighting Blindness.

REFERENCES

[1]   Dobell C, Leeuwenhoek Av. Antony van Leeuwenhoek and his "Little animals"; being some account of the father of protozoology and bacteriology and his multifarious discoveries in these disciplines. New York: Harcourt, Brace and company 1932. vii, 435, 1.

[2]   Nigg EA, Raff JW. Centrioles, centrosomes, and cilia in health and disease. Cell 2009; 139(4): 663-78. [http://dx.doi.org/10.1016/j.cell.2009.10.036] [PMID: 19914163]

[3]   Badano JL, Mitsuma N, Beales PL, Katsanis N. The ciliopathies: an emerging class of human genetic disorders. Annu Rev Genomics Hum Genet 2006; 7: 125-48. [http://dx.doi.org/10.1146/annurev.genom.7.080505.115610] [PMID: 16722803]

[4]   Berbari NF, O'Connor AK, Haycraft CJ, Yoder BK. The primary cilium as a complex signaling center. Curr Biol 2009; 19(13): R526-35. [http://dx.doi.org/10.1016/j.cub.2009.05.025] [PMID: 19602418]

[5]   Eggenschwiler JT, Anderson KV. Cilia and developmental signaling. Annu Rev Cell Dev Biol 2007; 23: 345-73. [http://dx.doi.org/10.1146/annurev.cellbio.23.090506.123249] [PMID: 17506691]

[6]   Singla V, Reiter JF. The primary cilium as the cell's antenna: signaling at a sensory organelle. Science 2006; 313(5787): 629-33. [http://dx.doi.org/10.1126/science.1124534] [PMID: 16888132]

[7]   Shah AS, Ben-Shahar Y, Moninger TO, Kline JN, Welsh MJ. Motile cilia of human airway epithelia are chemosensory. Science 2009; 325(5944): 1131-4.
[http://dx.doi.org/10.1126/science.1173869] [PMID: 19628819]

[8]   Anand M, Khanna H. Ciliary transition zone (TZ) proteins RPGR and CEP290: role in photoreceptor cilia and degenerative diseases. Expert Opin Ther Targets 2012; 16(6): 541-51.
[http://dx.doi.org/10.1517/14728222.2012.680956] [PMID: 22563985]

[9]   Yildiz O, Khanna H. Ciliary signaling cascades in photoreceptors. Vision Res 2012; 75: 112-6.
[http://dx.doi.org/10.1016/j.visres.2012.08.007] [PMID: 22921640]

[10]   Keady BT, Samtani R, Tobita K, *et al.* IFT25 links the signal-dependent movement of Hedgehog components to intraflagellar transport. Dev Cell 2012; 22(5): 940-51.
[http://dx.doi.org/10.1016/j.devcel.2012.04.009] [PMID: 22595669]

[11]   Cole DG. The intraflagellar transport machinery of Chlamydomonas reinhardtii. Traffic 2003; 4(7): 435-42.
[http://dx.doi.org/10.1034/j.1600-0854.2003.t01-1-00103.x] [PMID: 12795688]

[12]   Cole DG, Diener DR, Himelblau AL, Beech PL, Fuster JC, Rosenbaum JL. Chlamydomonas kinesin-II-dependent intraflagellar transport (IFT): IFT particles contain proteins required for ciliary assembly in Caenorhabditis elegans sensory neurons. J Cell Biol 1998; 141(4): 993-1008.
[http://dx.doi.org/10.1083/jcb.141.4.993] [PMID: 9585417]

[13]   Follit JA, Xu F, Keady BT, Pazour GJ. Characterization of mouse IFT complex B. Cell Motil Cytoskeleton 2009; 66(8): 457-68.
[http://dx.doi.org/10.1002/cm.20346] [PMID: 19253336]

[14]   Piperno G, Mead K. Transport of a novel complex in the cytoplasmic matrix of Chlamydomonas flagella. Proc Natl Acad Sci USA 1997; 94(9): 4457-62.
[http://dx.doi.org/10.1073/pnas.94.9.4457] [PMID: 9114011]

[15]   Storm van's Gravesande K, Omran H. Primary ciliary dyskinesia: clinical presentation, diagnosis and genetics. Ann Med 2005; 37(6): 439-49.
[http://dx.doi.org/10.1080/07853890510011985] [PMID: 16203616]

[16]   Afzelius BA. A human syndrome caused by immotile cilia. Science 1976; 193(4250): 317-9.
[http://dx.doi.org/10.1126/science.1084576] [PMID: 1084576]

[17]   Baccetti B, Afzelius BA. The biology of the sperm cell. Monogr Dev Biol 1976; (10): 1-254.
[PMID: 1107820]

[18]   Afzelius BA. Cilia-related diseases. J Pathol 2004; 204(4): 470-7.
[http://dx.doi.org/10.1002/path.1652] [PMID: 15495266]

[19]   Lamb TD. Evolution of phototransduction, vertebrate photoreceptors and retina. Prog Retin Eye Res 2013; 36: 52-119.
[http://dx.doi.org/10.1016/j.preteyeres.2013.06.001] [PMID: 23792002]

[20]   Besharse JC, Bok D. The retina and its disorders. Amsterdam ; Boston: Academic Press 2011. xvi, 912.

[21]   Dowling JE. The retina: an approachable part of the brain Rev ed. Cambridge, Mass: Belknap Press of Harvard University Press 2012. xvi, 355

[22]   Merbs SL, Nathans J. Absorption spectra of human cone pigments. Nature 1992; 356(6368): 433-5.
[http://dx.doi.org/10.1038/356433a0] [PMID: 1557124]

[23]   Nathans J. The genes for color vision. Sci Am 1989; 260(2): 42-9.
[http://dx.doi.org/10.1038/scientificamerican0289-42] [PMID: 2643825]

[24]   Nathans J. The evolution and physiology of human color vision: insights from molecular genetic studies of visual pigments. Neuron 1999; 24(2): 299-312.

[http://dx.doi.org/10.1016/S0896-6273(00)80845-4] [PMID: 10571225]

[25]   Remington LA, Remington LA. Clinical anatomy and physiology of the visual system. 3rd ed., St. Louis, Mo.: Elsevier/Butterworth Heinemann 2012. ix, 292.

[26]   Punzo C, Kornacker K, Cepko CL. Stimulation of the insulin/mTOR pathway delays cone death in a mouse model of retinitis pigmentosa. Nat Neurosci 2009; 12(1): 44-52.
        [http://dx.doi.org/10.1038/nn.2234] [PMID: 19060896]

[27]   Léveillard T, Mohand-Saïd S, Lorentz O, *et al.* Identification and characterization of rod-derived cone viability factor. Nat Genet 2004; 36(7): 755-9.
        [http://dx.doi.org/10.1038/ng1386] [PMID: 15220920]

[28]   Mears AJ, Kondo M, Swain PK, *et al.* Nrl is required for rod photoreceptor development. Nat Genet 2001; 29(4): 447-52.
        [http://dx.doi.org/10.1038/ng774] [PMID: 11694879]

[29]   Saade CJ, Alvarez-Delfin K, Fadool JM. Rod photoreceptors protect from cone degeneration-induced retinal remodeling and restore visual responses in zebrafish. J Neurosci 2013; 33(5): 1804-14.
        [http://dx.doi.org/10.1523/JNEUROSCI.2910-12.2013] [PMID: 23365220]

[30]   Kessel RG, Kardon RH. Tissues and organs: a text-atlas of scanning electron microscopy. San Francisco: W. H. Freeman 1979. ix, 317.

[31]   Peters KR, Palade GE, Schneider BG, Papermaster DS. Fine structure of a periciliary ridge complex of frog retinal rod cells revealed by ultrahigh resolution scanning electron microscopy. J Cell Biol 1983; 96(1): 265-76.
        [http://dx.doi.org/10.1083/jcb.96.1.265] [PMID: 6219117]

[32]   Liu X, Bulgakov OV, Darrow KN, *et al.* Usherin is required for maintenance of retinal photoreceptors and normal development of cochlear hair cells. Proc Natl Acad Sci USA 2007; 104(11): 4413-8.
        [http://dx.doi.org/10.1073/pnas.0610950104] [PMID: 17360538]

[33]   Maerker T, van Wijk E, Overlack N, *et al.* A novel Usher protein network at the periciliary reloading point between molecular transport machineries in vertebrate photoreceptor cells. Hum Mol Genet 2008; 17(1): 71-86.
        [http://dx.doi.org/10.1093/hmg/ddm285] [PMID: 17906286]

[34]   De Robertis E. Some observations on the ultrastructure and morphogenesis of photoreceptors. J Gen Physiol 1960; 43(6) (Suppl.): 1-13.
        [http://dx.doi.org/10.1085/jgp.43.6.1] [PMID: 13814989]

[35]   Cohen AI. Further studies on the question of the patency of saccules in outer segments of vertebrate photoreceptors. Vision Res 1970; 10(6): 445-53.
        [http://dx.doi.org/10.1016/0042-6989(70)90001-5] [PMID: 4099086]

[36]   Dowling JE. Foveal Receptors of the Monkey Retina: Fine Structure. Science 1965; 147(3653): 57-9.
        [http://dx.doi.org/10.1126/science.147.3653.57] [PMID: 14224526]

[37]   Chakraborty D, Conley SM, Stuck MW, Naash MI. Differences in RDS trafficking, assembly and function in cones *versus* rods: insights from studies of C150S-RDS. Hum Mol Genet 2010; 19(24): 4799-812.
        [http://dx.doi.org/10.1093/hmg/ddq410] [PMID: 20858597]

[38]   Cheng T, Peachey NS, Li S, Goto Y, Cao Y, Naash MI. The effect of peripherin/rds haploinsufficiency on rod and cone photoreceptors. J Neurosci 1997; 17(21): 8118-28.
        [PMID: 9334387]

[39]   Farjo R, Fliesler SJ, Naash MI. Effect of Rds abundance on cone outer segment morphogenesis, photoreceptor gene expression, and outer limiting membrane integrity. J Comp Neurol 2007; 504(6): 619-30.
        [http://dx.doi.org/10.1002/cne.21476] [PMID: 17722028]

[40]   Farjo R, Skaggs JS, Nagel BA, *et al.* Retention of function without normal disc morphogenesis occurs in cone but not rod photoreceptors. J Cell Biol 2006; 173(1): 59-68.
[http://dx.doi.org/10.1083/jcb.200509036] [PMID: 16585269]

[41]   Liu X, Wu TH, Stowe S, *et al.* Defective phototransductive disk membrane morphogenesis in transgenic mice expressing opsin with a mutated N-terminal domain. J Cell Sci 1997; 110(Pt 20): 2589-97.
[PMID: 9372448]

[42]   Skiba NP, Spencer WJ, Salinas RY, Lieu EC, Thompson JW, Arshavsky VY. Proteomic identification of unique photoreceptor disc components reveals the presence of PRCD, a protein linked to retinal degeneration. J Proteome Res 2013; 12(6): 3010-8.
[http://dx.doi.org/10.1021/pr4003678] [PMID: 23672200]

[43]   Besharse JC. A Model for Cell Biological Studies Part I. 3rd ed. New York: Academic Press 1986; pp. 297-352.

[44]   Wang J, Deretic D. Molecular complexes that direct rhodopsin transport to primary cilia. Prog Retin Eye Res 2014; 38: 1-19.
[http://dx.doi.org/10.1016/j.preteyeres.2013.08.004] [PMID: 24135424]

[45]   Aveldaño MI, Bazán NG. Molecular species of phosphatidylcholine, -ethanolamine, -serine, and -inositol in microsomal and photoreceptor membranes of bovine retina. J Lipid Res 1983; 24(5): 620-7.
[PMID: 6875386]

[46]   Rajala A, Dighe R, Agbaga MP, Anderson RE, Rajala RV. Insulin receptor signaling in cones. J Biol Chem 2013; 288(27): 19503-15.
[http://dx.doi.org/10.1074/jbc.M113.469064] [PMID: 23673657]

[47]   Winkler BS. An hypothesis to account for the renewal of outer segments in rod and cone photoreceptor cells: renewal as a surrogate antioxidant. Invest Ophthalmol Vis Sci 2008; 49(8): 3259-61.
[http://dx.doi.org/10.1167/iovs.08-1785] [PMID: 18660422]

[48]   Young RW. The renewal of photoreceptor cell outer segments. J Cell Biol 1967; 33(1): 61-72.
[http://dx.doi.org/10.1083/jcb.33.1.61] [PMID: 6033942]

[49]   Bok D, Young RW. The renewal of diffusely distributed protein in the outer segments of rods and cones. Vision Res 1972; 12(2): 161-8.
[http://dx.doi.org/10.1016/0042-6989(72)90108-3] [PMID: 4537522]

[50]   Steinberg RH, Fisher SK, Anderson DH. Disc morphogenesis in vertebrate photoreceptors. J Comp Neurol 1980; 190(3): 501-8.
[http://dx.doi.org/10.1002/cne.901900307] [PMID: 6771304]

[51]   Matsumoto B, Besharse JC. Light and temperature modulated staining of the rod outer segment distal tips with Lucifer yellow. Invest Ophthalmol Vis Sci 1985; 26(5): 628-35.
[PMID: 2581915]

[52]   Chuang JZ, Zhao Y, Sung CH. SARA-regulated vesicular targeting underlies formation of the light-sensing organelle in mammalian rods. Cell 2007; 130(3): 535-47.
[http://dx.doi.org/10.1016/j.cell.2007.06.030] [PMID: 17693260]

[53]   Sung CH, Chuang JZ. The cell biology of vision. J Cell Biol 2010; 190(6): 953-63.
[http://dx.doi.org/10.1083/jcb.201006020] [PMID: 20855501]

[54]   Gilliam JC, Chang JT, Sandoval IM, *et al.* Three-dimensional architecture of the rod sensory cilium and its disruption in retinal neurodegeneration. Cell 2012; 151(5): 1029-41.
[http://dx.doi.org/10.1016/j.cell.2012.10.038] [PMID: 23178122]

[55]   Burgoyne T, Meschede IP, Burden JJ, Bailly M, Seabra MC, Futter CE. Rod disc renewal occurs by evagination of the ciliary plasma membrane that makes cadherin-based contacts with the inner

segment. Proc Natl Acad Sci USA 2015; 112(52): 15922-7.
[http://dx.doi.org/10.1073/pnas.1509285113] [PMID: 26668363]

[56]   Volland S, Hughes LC, Kong C, *et al.* Three-dimensional organization of nascent rod outer segment disk membranes. Proc Natl Acad Sci USA 2015; 112(48): 14870-5.
[http://dx.doi.org/10.1073/pnas.1516309112] [PMID: 26578801]

[57]   Pugh EN Jr. Photoreceptor disc morphogenesis: The classical evagination model prevails. J Cell Biol 2015; 211(3): 491-3.
[http://dx.doi.org/10.1083/jcb.201510067] [PMID: 26527745]

[58]   Travis GH, Golczak M, Moise AR, Palczewski K. Diseases caused by defects in the visual cycle: retinoids as potential therapeutic agents. Annu Rev Pharmacol Toxicol 2007; 47: 469-512.
[http://dx.doi.org/10.1146/annurev.pharmtox.47.120505.105225] [PMID: 16968212]

[59]   Luo DG, Xue T, Yau KW. How vision begins: an odyssey. Proc Natl Acad Sci USA 2008; 105(29): 9855-62.
[http://dx.doi.org/10.1073/pnas.0708405105] [PMID: 18632568]

[60]   Kim YK, Kim JH, Yu YS, Ko HW, Kim JH. Localization of primary cilia in mouse retina. Acta Histochem 2013; 115(8): 789-94.
[http://dx.doi.org/10.1016/j.acthis.2013.03.005] [PMID: 23608602]

[61]   Ferraro S, Gomez-Montalvo AI, Olmos R, Ramirez M, Lamas M. Primary cilia in rat mature Müller glia: downregulation of IFT20 expression reduces sonic hedgehog-mediated proliferation and dedifferentiation potential of Müller glia primary cultures. Cell Mol Neurobiol 2015; 35(4): 533-42.
[http://dx.doi.org/10.1007/s10571-014-0149-3] [PMID: 25504432]

[62]   Kim J, Lee JE, Heynen-Genel S, *et al.* Functional genomic screen for modulators of ciliogenesis and cilium length. Nature 2010; 464(7291): 1048-51.
[http://dx.doi.org/10.1038/nature08895] [PMID: 20393563]

[63]   Nishiyama K, Sakaguchi H, Hu JG, Bok D, Hollyfield JG. Claudin localization in cilia of the retinal pigment epithelium. Anat Rec 2002; 267(3): 196-203.
[http://dx.doi.org/10.1002/ar.10102] [PMID: 12115268]

[64]   Klagsbrun M, D'Amore PA. Angiogenesis: biology and pathology. Cold Spring Harbor, N.Y.: Cold Spring Harbor Laboratory Press 2012. xiv, 522

[65]   Egorova AD, Khedoe PP, Goumans MJ, *et al.* Lack of primary cilia primes shear-induced endothelial-to-mesenchymal transition. Circ Res 2011; 108(9): 1093-101.
[http://dx.doi.org/10.1161/CIRCRESAHA.110.231860] [PMID: 21393577]

[66]   Luo N, Conwell MD, Chen X, *et al.* Primary cilia signaling mediates intraocular pressure sensation. Proc Natl Acad Sci USA 2014; 111(35): 12871-6.
[http://dx.doi.org/10.1073/pnas.1323292111] [PMID: 25143588]

[67]   Blitzer AL, Panagis L, Gusella GL, Danias J, Mlodzik M, Iomini C. Primary cilia dynamics instruct tissue patterning and repair of corneal endothelium. Proc Natl Acad Sci USA 2011; 108(7): 2819-24.
[http://dx.doi.org/10.1073/pnas.1016702108] [PMID: 21285373]

CHAPTER 2

Zebrafish Models of Photoreceptor Ciliopathies

Brian D. Perkins[*]

Department of Ophthalmic Research, Cole Eye Institute, Cleveland Clinic, 9500 Euclid Ave. Cleveland, OH 44195, USA

Abstract: Ciliopathies refer to a genetically and clinically heterogeneous class of disorders that result from defects in the formation or function of the primary cilium. Cilia are the microtubule-based organelles that protrude from the surface of almost all vertebrate cells, including the rod and cone photoreceptors. The photoreceptor sensory cilium consists of the connecting cilium and outer segment with the outer segment forming a unique structure containing thousands of tightly packed disc membranes. Mutations in over 50 genes result in syndromic ciliopathies that can manifest with retinal degeneration, including Bardet-Biedl syndrome (BBS), Joubert Syndrome, Jeune Syndrome, and nephronophthisis (NPHP) or in non-syndromic retinal dystrophies like Leber Congenital Amaurosis (LCA) and Retinitis Pigmentosa (RP). Zebrafish have been widely used as a model system to study ciliopathies, particularly BBS and Joubert Syndrome, and for studying the mechanisms leading to photoreceptor degeneration associated with these disorders. Investigators were drawn to zebrafish due to the rapid growth and transparency of the zebrafish embryo, the differentiation of photoreceptors by 3 days post-fertilization, and the ability to suppress gene function through morpholino knockdown. The genetic heterogeneity of ciliopathies and desire for more accurate genotype-phenotype correlations make zebrafish an appealing model for studying gene- and allele-specific differences in a rapid manner. This review will discuss the current zebrafish models of retinal ciliopathies, evaluate the widespread use of morpholinos as tools to knock down gene function in zebrafish, and make predictions on how zebrafish will contribute in future studies of ciliopathies.

Keywords: *ahi1*, *arl13b*, Bardet-Biedl Syndrome, BBS, *cep290*, Ciliopathies, Cilium, Joubert Syndrome, Photoreceptor, Retina, Retinal Degeneration, Sensory Cilium, Zebrafish.

INTRODUCTION

Cilia are microtubule-based organelles that typically project from the apical surface of almost all vertebrate cells and remain surrounded by the plasma membrane. At the base of each cilium is a protein and microtubule-based structure

[*] **Corresponding author Brian D. Perkins:** Cole Eye Institute, 9500 Euclid Ave. Cleveland, OH, USA; Tel: 216-444-9683; E-mail: perkinb2@ccf.org

Hemant Khanna (Ed)

called the basal body. The basal body is a modified centriole that nucleates cilium formation and serves to link the cilium with the rest of the cytoskeleton. Ciliary microtubules organize in pairs to form an axoneme, the structural backbone of the cilium. The axoneme is organized with either a "9+2" or "9+0" geometry, depending on the presence of a central pair of microtubule doublets, although exceptions to these rules do exist [1]. Motile cilia typically have a "9+2" axoneme, while non-motile and primary cilia possess a "9+0" axoneme. For many years, research in cilia largely focused on the role of cilia in cellular locomotion in single-cell eukaryotes and in fluid movement in certain tissues. In the early 2000s, however, interest in ciliary biology exploded when genes encoding cilia or basal body proteins were directly linked to the multi-syndromic diseases termed "ciliopathies". The ciliopathies exhibit a variety of clinical symptoms that typically involve kidney, eye, brain, and skeletal abnormalities, along with other variable phenotypes [2, 3]. To better understand the role of cilia in development and the etiology of disease, scientists often turned to zebrafish as an *in vivo* model to study cilia pathology. Forward genetic screens in zebrafish identified mutations in cilia-related genes, but morpholino oligonucleotides were widely used to knock-down gene function. Since 2004, cilia have been the subject of almost 800 review articles discussing the role of cilia in signaling [4 - 8], development [9, 10], and disease [2, 3, 11], as well perspectives on trafficking mechanisms and motors in cilia [12 - 14], and cilia evolution [15, 16]. With so many authoritative and exhaustive reviews available, it would seem redundant to address these topics again. Missing from these commentaries, however, is a closer inspection of the tools, techniques, and experimental approaches taken when using zebrafish as a model, as well as the resulting phenotypes. In light of new advances with genome editing tools, such as TALE nucleases (TALENs) and CRISPRs, it would be useful to catalog the phenotypes reported for zebrafish cilia mutants and phenotypes obtained from morpholino injections and consider commonalities and differences in these phenotypes. This review will describe the photoreceptor sensory cilium, provide a brief overview of ciliopathy diseases, and finally, examine how researchers have used the zebrafish as a model to understand the genetics and cell biology of ciliopathies, with a particular emphasis on photoreceptors.

The Photoreceptor Sensory Cilium

Vertebrate photoreceptors consist of a light-sensitive outer segment, an inner segment containing the biosynthetic machinery, and a synaptic terminal. The photoreceptor outer segments contain hundreds of tightly stacked disc membranes, with each disc membrane containing thousands of molecules of the visual pigment and the machinery for phototransduction. The visual pigment of rods is the G-protein coupled receptor rhodopsin, while cones express specific cone opsins with sensitivities to different wavelengths of light. It is estimated that an individual photoreceptor contains approximately one billion opsin molecules, in addition to components of the G-protein cascade necessary for light detection. Protein synthesis, however, occurs in the inner segment and a highly efficient trafficking mechanism transports proteins to the outer segment. The inner and outer segments are connected by a thin, nonmotile cilium. First identified as a bona fide ciliary structure by electron microscopy in 1956 by Eduardo De Robertis [17], the photoreceptor connecting cilium was considered distinct from the outer segment and largely regarded as little more than a passageway for phototransduction proteins destined for the outer segment. Today, the connecting cilium and outer segment are together considered a single "sensory cilium" with a ciliary proteome consisting of almost 2000 proteins [18].

Photoreceptor sensory cilia exhibit many characteristics typical of all cilia, as well as a number of features unique to photoreceptors. The structure of photoreceptor cilia has been studied for years by electron microscopy [17, 19, 20], as well as by freeze-fracture analysis [21], and recently by cryo-electron tomography [22]. Like all cilia, photoreceptor sensory cilia contain an axoneme, a transition zone (*i.e.* the connecting cilium), and a basal body anchoring the cilium to the cytoskeleton by a long, striated rootlet [22]. Photoreceptors contain two basal bodies. The distal basal body, or mother centriole, sits at the top of the rootlet and serves as a template for the microtubule doublets of the axoneme. The proximal basal body, or daughter centriole, aligns perpendicularly with the distal basal body but does not generate an axoneme. Microtubule triplets project apically from the distal basal body and transition into doublets to form the 9+0 nonmotile axoneme, which extends through the transition zone (*i.e.* connecting cilium) and into the outer segment. The microtubule doublets split apart within the distal outer segment and extend to the outer segment tips as microtubule singlets in both mammals and zebrafish [23, 24]. The most distinctive, and unique, feature of the photoreceptor cilium is the massive volume occupied by the disc membranes. Like other primary cilia, the process of Intraflagellar Transport (IFT) is required for the development and maintenance of the photoreceptor connecting cilium and outer segment [24 - 30]. The details of IFT [12, 31], the IFT motors [13, 14, 32], its requirements for photoreceptor sensory cilia [33, 34] have been extensively reviewed elsewhere and interested readers are encouraged to seek out these sources.

The anatomical structure of the photoreceptor cilium and molecular mechanisms governing cilia development and maintenance are highly conserved among vertebrates. As this review focuses on zebrafish, however, a few key distinctions between zebrafish, rodent, and human photoreceptor sensory cilia should be briefly mentioned. First, calyceal processes are present in the photoreceptors of primates, zebrafish and other non-mammalian vertebrates, but are absent in mice [35, 36]. Calyceal processes are microvilli-like structures made up of actin filaments, which radiate axially in a parallel fashion from the inner segment and extend to form a collar around the base of the outer segment. The function of the calyceal processes is unclear, but recent evidence demonstrated that the Usher 1 proteins myosin VIIa, harmonin, and cadherin-23 localize to these structures in humans [35], which may have implications in the pathophysiology of Usher Syndrome. Second, zebrafish have cone-dominated retinas, whereas mice are rod dominated (95-97% rods) and humans are rod-dominated with a cone-rich fovea. Zebrafish possess four cone subtypes that are sensitive to UV, blue, green, and red light. These photoreceptors express cone subtype-specific opsins and organize in a highly-ordered row mosaic [37, 38]. Finally, the cone sensory cilia also exhibit exquisite planar polarity. In flat-mounts of adult zebrafish retinas, the basal bodies of the blue-, red-, and green-sensitive cones can be observed to orient on one side of the inner segment and align towards the optic nerve [39]. It is not clear whether basal bodies in rodent photoreceptors share this asymmetrical arrangement, but evidence from tree shrews suggested that a similar planar alignment of basal bodies and connecting cilia occurs in a primate-like species [40].

Ciliopathies

Ciliopathies refer to a spectrum of human syndromes that are attributed to defects in either motile cilia, non-motile cilia, or both [2, 3, 41]. The first description of a disease now known to be a ciliopathy appeared in the 1930s by Kartagener [42]. Bardet-Biedl Syndrome (BBS) [43] and Joubert Syndrome (JBST) [44] were identified by distinct clinical classifications more than 40 years ago. In 1976, Afzelius was the first to directly link defects in motile cilia with a human syndrome, which was characterized by bronchitis, immotile sperm, and sinusitis [45]. As diagnostic criteria grew more specific and additional pleiotropic syndromes were identified, more than a dozen syndromes became recognized as ciliopathies, including JBTS, BBS, Meckle-Gruber Syndrome, Alstrom Syndrome, nephronophthisis, and Senior-Loken Syndrome [2]. These syndromes have distinct clinical classifications but many diagnostic phenotypes, including kidney cysts, mental retardation, polydactyly, skeletal defects, and retinal degeneration, overlap or show variable penetrance. Throughout the 1990s, genetic screens in species ranging from *Chlamydomonas* [46 - 50] to *C. elegans* [51, 52] to zebrafish [53] and mice [54 - 57] began identifying mutants with defects in cilia. Subsequent biochemical studies revealed that the mutated genes encoded proteins that localized to basal bodies and cilia. With the release of completed genome sequences for various organisms, including humans, it became apparent that many of the human syndromes were caused by mutations in genes encoding proteins associated with the basal body or cilium. Today, more than 50 genes have been identified that cause ciliopathies.

Visual deficits are routinely included in the list of symptoms for most ciliopathies. Genetic mutations affecting cilia form or function most likely result in photoreceptor degeneration, typically in the form of retinitis pigmentosa (RP). When diagnosed in younger children, the diagnosis is often Leber Congenital Amaurosis (LCA). The location of photoreceptor degeneration varies within the retina and no clear-cut pattern exists. Photoreceptor loss can occur in either the periphery or in the central retina and both rod-cone and cone-rod dystrophies have been reported for BBS patients, based on fundus examinations and electroretinogram (ERG) recordings [58 - 60]. Retinal degeneration is also reported for JBST patients, but other ocular abnormalities can also exist [61]. In a survey of 8 JBST children, with ages ranging from 7 months to 10 years, only 3 patients had findings of retinal dystrophy and none had yet developed abnormal ERGs [61]. Common findings were defects in saccades, nystagmus, and strabismus [61, 62]. While a percentage of JBST patients have subnormal ERGs thresholds, such deficits do not appear to be a universal clinical finding [63, 64]. Visual defects have also been reported for patients with Senior-Loken Syndrome and Jeune Syndrome, although the degree of pathology varies between different syndromes [65, 66]. Such differences likely reflect differences in gene mutations, modifiers, and triallelism [67, 68]. The retinal pathology in these various disorders exhibits a high degree of heterogeneity, making genotype-phenotype correlations more difficult. This prompted investigators to conduct studies in genetically tractable model organisms.

ZEBRAFISH MODELS OF CILIOPATHIES

To better understand the molecular mechanisms leading to pathology in ciliopathies, investigators quickly utilized zebrafish to model the disease state. As a vertebrate, the physiology, biochemistry and anatomy of the zebrafish retina, kidney, and nervous system share a number of similarities to humans. The rapid embryonic development of zebrafish, the relatively low expense of maintaining a small zebrafish colony, and expanding infrastructure in genomics and molecular tools combined to make zebrafish an attractive model. In the early 1990s, large-scale forward genetic screens of chemically-mutagenized fish identified hundreds of mutants [69, 70], including several that possessed multi-organ phenotypes similar to that of ciliopathies [71, 72]. Following gene identification by positional cloning, it became apparent that the mutated genes encoded IFT proteins [27, 73, 74], ciliary motors [75], tubulin modifying enzymes [76], and orthologs to human disease genes [73, 77]. For dozens of other genes, antisense morpholino oligonucleotides (MOs) were used to selectively "knock-down" the function of zebrafish orthologs to generate phenotypes [78 - 91]. The use of morpholinos spread rapidly as a strategy for reverse-genetics. Targeted gene deletion *via* homologous recombination (*i.e.* "knock-out" technology), which is a staple of mouse genetics, relies on embryonic stem cells and has not successfully translated to zebrafish. In contrast, morpholinos generate loss-of-function effects for any gene of interest, the morpholino-injected embryos (*i.e.* "morphants") can be scored for phenotypes of interest within the first 5 days post fertilization (dpf), and the morpholinos and microinjection equipment is affordable for individual laboratories.

Intraflagellar Transport (IFT) Mutants – The Gold Standard for Ciliopathy Phenotypes

The first zebrafish models to link defects in cilia with retinal degeneration and kidney cysts were the zebrafish *ift57*, *ift88* and *ift172* mutants [27, 73, 92]. These mutants were initially identified in forward genetic screens for recessive mutations resulting in eye- or kidney-specific phenotypes. Each gene encodes a component of the IFT particle, a multi-protein complex that mediates cargo trafficking through the cilium [12]. By 5 dpf, each mutant shows a common "ciliopathy" phenotype, consisting of kidney cysts, photoreceptor degeneration, and a ventral curvature of the tail and lethality by 8-9 dpf, phenotypes which can be readily scored under a stereomicroscope. The retinal phenotype of each mutant is extremely similar. All mutants undergo rapid photoreceptor degeneration and rods and cones are equally affected [27, 93]. Basal body positioning is unaffected, but the photoreceptor axoneme fails to form and outer segments are missing from the *ift88* and *ift172* mutants [93]. In contrast, the *ift57* mutants produce short outer segments. In the absence of the Ift57 protein, the kinesin-II motor fails to dissociate from the IFT particle and post-Golgi vesicles accumulate at the base of the cilium, suggesting that loss of Ift57 lowers the affinity of the IFT particle to rhodopsin-bound vesicles or reduced the efficiency of IFT particle recycling [29]. In all three mutants, opsins accumulates in the photoreceptor inner segment.

The zebrafish IFT mutants were the first vertebrate models to harbor complete loss-of-function mutations in an IFT component and to completely lack cilia. A hypomorphic mutation in the mouse *Ift88* gene, also known as *Tg737*, was identified in the *Oak Ridge Polycystic Kidney* (*orpk*) disease mouse model [94]. This mutant has kidney cysts and progressive photoreceptor degeneration and loss of outer segments [26]. The zebrafish *ift88* and *ift172* mutants, however, show a complete absence of outer segments or ciliary axonemes [27, 29, 93], reinforcing the model that IFT is essential for cilia formation and that this process is evolutionarily conserved from single-cell organisms through vertebrates. As loss of IFT results in the most direct and severe consequences on cilia formation, the associated cystic kidney and body curvature phenotypes of the IFT mutants became a convenient method to visually assess cilia abnormalities in zebrafish.

Zebrafish Models of Bardet-Biedl Syndrome (BBS)

The link between cilia dysfunction and multisystemic disease is perhaps best illustrated by Bardet-Biedl Syndrome (BBS), a ciliopathy that presents with a constellation of clinical features. The hallmarks of BBS are retinal degeneration, obesity, polydactyly, hypogonadism, kidney dysfunction, and mental retardation, with secondary features possibly including speech difficulties, diabetes and metabolic defects, and abnormalities affecting the hepatic, cardiovascular, and auditory systems [95]. Mutations in at least 19 distinct genes (*BBS1-19*) cause autosomal recessive BBS. Some forms of BBS also require an additional mutation in a third allele, indicating "triallelic inheritance" [68] or the need for a modifier allele [96]. While most patients with *BBS* gene mutations exhibit classic BBS symptoms, some recent clinical studies have reported *BBS* mutations in patients presenting with nonsyndromic RP [97 - 100]. Nonsense mutations in *bbs1*, *bbs2*, *bbs4*, *bbs7*, *bbs9*, *bbs11* (known as *trim32*), *bbs12*, *bbs13* (known as *mkks*), and *bbs14* (known as *cep290*) have been recovered in the Zebrafish Mutation Project at the Sanger Institute, but phenotypic descriptions of these mutants have not yet been reported (www.zfin.org). Morpholinos have been used to target *bbs1-14* [80 - 82, 101 - 105], and *bbs18* [106], but different groups have reported differing morphant phenotypes when targeting the same *bbs* gene. This variance may reflect morpholino sequence differences or the choice of phenotypes to report. Unfortunately, interpretations of morpholino phenotypes, particularly those related to *bbs* function, have recently come under increased scrutiny due to potential off-target effects [107].

Work from multiple groups has shown that suppressing *bbs* gene function can lead to cilia defects in certain cases. Kupffer's vesicle (KV) is a ciliated organ in zebrafish that is analogous to the embryonic node in mice. KV cilia function is required to establish left-right asymmetry. KV cilia are significantly shorter and fewer in number in *bbs2*, *bbs4, bbs5*, *bbs6*, *bbs7*and *bbs8* morphants, which results in laterality defects [82]. These morphants also exhibit defects in intracellular trafficking. In response to light or hormones, the melanosomes in the zebrafish skin will quickly aggregate near the nucleus by shuttling along microtubules in a dynein-dependent manner. The *bbs* morphants show significant delays in melanosome aggregation, suggesting a defect in retrograde trafficking. Retina phenotypes differ between various *bbs* morphants from these groups. Knockdown of *bbs7* does not cause any obvious effects on photoreceptor morphology [82]. Humans, mice, and zebrafish all express a retina-specific isoform of *BBS3*, called *BBS3L*, which differs from *BBS3* in the C-terminus [108]. Morpholinos specifically targeting *bbs3L* caused visual behavior defects and mild mislocalization of cone opsins that could was rescued by mRNA encoding human *BBS3L*, but not *BBS3* [108]. Finally, morpholino knockdown of *bbs4* cause partial mislocalization of rhodopsin and evidence of photoreceptor death, phenotypes which can be rescued by co-injecting mRNA encoding human *BBS4* [109]. Kidney cysts and a ventral body curvature are hallmark phenotypes of zebrafish cilia mutants, but only *bbs4* morphants show mild body curvature defects [110] and evidence for kidney cysts have not been reported for any *bbs* morphant.

Numerous studies by Katsanis and colleagues have reported that knockdown of *bbs* genes result in phenotypes that resemble defects in Planar Cell Polarity (PCP) [80, 81, 101, 104, 111]. In vertebrates, PCP regulates the collective cell migration, called convergent extension, during gastrulation [112 - 114] and also plays a role in the asymmetric localization of structures, like cilia, along a cell surface [115, 116]. The relationship between cilia and PCP signaling has been particularly confusing [7] and comes down to a chicken-or-the-egg question: does PCP signaling require cilia or does cilia formation require PCP? Morpholino knockdown of *bbs* genes result in convergent extension defects such as shortened body axes, broadened somites, and kinked notochords. This was complemented by reports that mouse mutants of *Bbs1*, *Bbs4*, and *Bbs6* exhibited disorganized stereocilia in the inner ear, which is a feature of PCP [81]. In addition, mouse and zebrafish mutants genetically interact with PCP genes like Vangl2 [81, 104, 117, 118]. In contrast, components of the PCP pathway are required to establish normal rotation of motile cilia in the neural tube [119], as well as normal basal body docking and ciliogenesis in *Xenopus* [115, 120]. This suggests PCP signaling acts upstream to regulate proper ciliogenesis. It has been argued that defective PCP signaling may contribute to the neural tube closure abnormalities, hearing loss, and the renal cysts that occur in BBS patients [81, 103, 121]. PCP defects, however, do not appear in zebrafish with genetic mutations in genes functioning in cilia formation, such as the *ift* genes (Fig. **1**); and [27, 73, 107]. This has led some to question whether the gastrulation phenotypes of *bbs* morphants reflect nonspecific effects of the morpholinos [107]. Alternatively, Bbs proteins may play cilia-independent roles in PCP signaling, or that the basal body and cilium should be considered distinct organelles and PCP signaling only requires the basal body [122, 123]. Such questions are unlikely to be resolved until zebrafish *bbs* genetic mutants have been thoroughly characterized.

Zebrafish Models of Joubert Syndrome

Joubert Syndrome (JBTS) represents a spectrum of disorders characterized primarily by hypoplasia of the cerebellar vermis, which appears as a "molar tooth sign" by magnetic resonance imaging (MRI) with variable degrees of retinal degeneration, hypotonia, ataxia, learning disabilities, and other cilia defects [124].

Like BBS, JBTS exhibits considerable genetic heterogeneity and perhaps even greater clinical variability. To date, mutations in 22 genes are known to cause JBTS and all function at the cilium. Of these, mutations in the *cc2d2a* and *arl13b* genes have been described in zebrafish [73, 77]. Nonsense mutations in *cep290*, *kif7*, and *tmem67* have been recovered in the Zebrafish Mutation Project at the Sanger Institute, but descriptions of these have not yet been reported (www.zfin.org). Finally, morpholino knockdowns have been conducted for zebrafish orthologs of *pde6d, csppl, cep41, tmem237, ttc21b, nphp1, ahi1, tmem216* [88 - 90, 125 - 129].

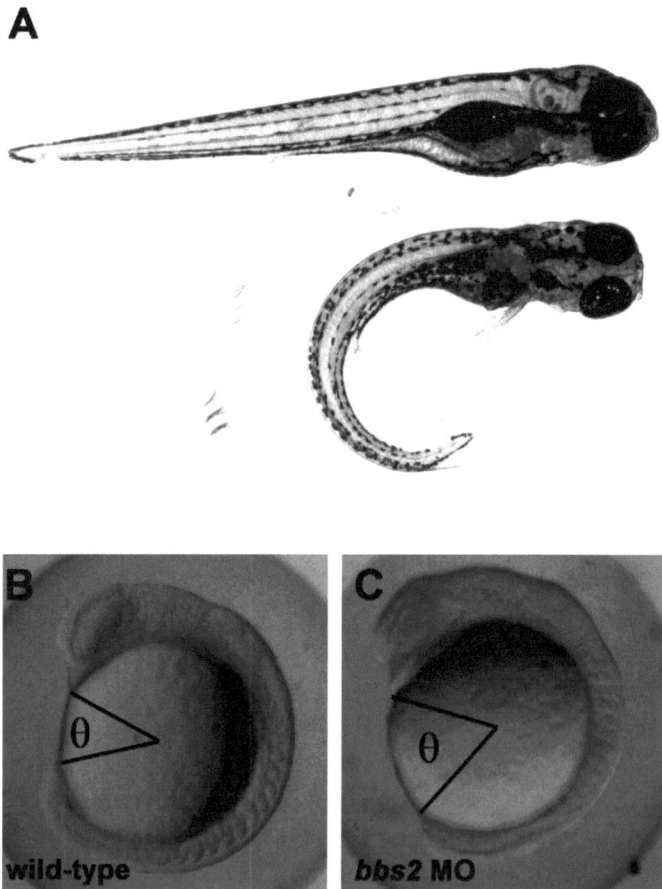

Fig. (1). Phenotypes of zebrafish ciliopathy mutants and morphants.
(A). Lateral view of wild-type (top) and *ift57* morphant (bottom) at 5 dpf. The curved tail and lack of swim bladder are readily observable phenotypes. **(B)** Lateral view of a wild-type embryo at 10-12 somite stage. The gap angle between the head and tail (θ) can be used to assess convergent-extension movements. **(C)** In a *bbs2* morphant, defects in cell migration during convergent-extension movements in gastrulation lead to a wider gap angle and a shortened body axis. This phenotype has been observed for many *bbs* morphants but not in *ift* mutants.

The zebrafish *cc2d2a* mutant was originally identified as a novel gene in a screen for modulators of mechanosensory hair cell death [130] and was subsequently shown to have kidney cysts [131]. After realizing the *cc2d2a* gene causes JBTS in humans, the zebrafish mutant was shown to also genetically interact with *cep290* to enhance the cystic kidney phenotype, reinforcing the hypothesis that *cc2d2a* is critical for cilia function [131]. In the retina, loss of *cc2d2a* results in defects in outer segment morphogenesis, attenuation of the photopic ERG waveform, and vesicle accumulation within the inner segment [77]. Multiple lines of evidence point to Cc2d2a functioning to regulate ciliary entry. Cc2d2a localizes to the ciliary transition zone and forms a complex with TMEM231 and B9D1 to function as a diffusion barrier into the ciliary membrane [132]. In *cc2d2a* mutants, Rab8 localization is also abnormal. Collectively, these results suggest that Cc2d2a functions in a larger complex to prevent diffusion and/or facilitate Rab8-mediated ciliary entry of cargo-containing post-Golgi vesicles.

The zebrafish *arl13b* mutant was identified from a large-scale insertional mutagenesis screen of ~450 lines for kidney cyst mutants [73, 133]. Zebrafish *arl13b* mutants exhibit a similar ventral body curvature and kidney cysts that resemble the *ift* mutant phenotype and the mutants die by 9 dpf [134]. Cilia numbers are reduced in *arl13b* mutants and ciliary motility is reduced. The axoneme structure, however, remains largely intact in the surviving cilia. When this collection of insertional mutants was also screened for ocular phenotypes, the *ift57* and *ift172* mutants were also identified but not *arl13b* [92], suggesting that loss of *arl13b* may not affect the retina. Work from my lab has found that loss of *arl13b* causes a small reduction in outer segment length during larval stages and slow photoreceptor degeneration over the course of weeks (unpublished observations).

Phenotypes of zebrafish morphants vary considerably and different assays have been used to model JBTS in zebrafish, although ocular phenotypes are rarely described. Injection of *pde6d* morpholinos result in hydrocephalus, kidney cysts, and retinal abnormalities [135]. At 3 dpf, the *pde6d* morphant retinas show defects in retinal lamination and apoptosis throughout the retina. These phenotypes can be partially rescued by wild-type mRNA. The mechanistic links between *pde6d*, cilia, and retinal lamination are not entirely clear, but retinal dysplasia and lamination defects were seen in histopathology of a deceased JBTS patient with homozygous *PDE6D* mutations, indicating that the lamination defect was not due to nonspecific effects of the morpholino [125]. Knockdown of *ahi1* causes a dorsal tail curvature, hydrocephalus, kidney cysts, and small eyes. Retinal histology was not described, but injection of wild-type *ahi1* mRNA could rescue these phenotypes [129]. Morphants of *cspp1a* were shown to have kidney cysts, hydrocephalus, heart edema and skeletal abnormalities, which are all common phenotypes to JBTS or other ciliopathies [126]. Similarly, *cep41* morphants also showed pericardial edema and hydrocephalus [90]. Knockdown of *tmem237*, *nphp1*, and *ttc21b* was shown to result in the PCP-like gastrulation phenotypes by 12 hpf [89, 127, 128].

The Mutant *vs.* Morphant Controversy

Morpholino technology has significantly influenced how zebrafish are utilized for scientific research. Prior to the introduction of morpholinos [136], assessing loss-of-function phenotypes in zebrafish could only be done in genetic mutants identified in forward genetic screens. Several hundred mutants were identified by a variety of screening approaches [69, 70, 133, 137, 138]. The advantage of screening for mutants with a given phenotype is that researchers were unbiased with respect to the loci required for a given process. This approach uncovered novel genes, as well as assigned new functions to previously known genes. The downside was that the screens were exceedingly time- and labor-intensive, the screens did not reach saturation, and identifying the mutated gene required positional cloning, which carried its own set of challenges. With morpholinos, however, researchers could quickly knockdown any gene of interest for functional studies and no longer relied on the availability of a mutant.

Recently, the use of morpholinos has come under heightened scrutiny and there is rapidly growing skepticism over morpholino specificity and the future use of morpholinos. Despite evidence of off-target effects, efforts to codify the standards for control experiments when using morpholinos have been largely unsuccessful or unevenly applied [139]. Many papers report injecting increasing doses of morpholinos until a "desired phenotype" is achieved, rather than entertaining the possibility that such phenotypes may not reflect the true function of the gene. It seems important to compare the morphant phenotype with the phenotypes of mouse knockouts or symptoms of human disease and consider off-target effects. Many of the reported morphant phenotypes would be easily identified in genetic screens, so it is curious why so few ciliopathy loci were identified in large-scale mutagenesis projects. Morphant phenotypes are rarely 100% penetrant and attempts to rescue the phenotypes by injecting wild-type RNA typically fail to rescue all the morphants. Perhaps most concerning, a recent study found that more than 80% of morphant phenotypes could not observed in the corresponding genetic mutant [140].

New reverse genetic technologies have created another paradigm shift for the zebrafish research community. Transcription activator-like effector nucleases (TALENs) [141, 142] and the CRISPR/Cas9 system [143, 144] now enable researchers to generate targeted mutations in any gene of interest in zebrafish.

TALENs and CRISPRs show tremendous promise and have been embraced by the zebrafish community. It is now possible to generate insertion/deletion mutations that destroy the function of a gene, to generate targeted mutations that correspond to human disease alleles, and even generate targeted conditional alleles [141]. As CRISPR technology improves, it has become possible to inject multiple CRISPR single guide RNAs (sgRNAs) to "multiplex" screen the CRISPR injected animals for loss-of-function phenotypes prior to establishing germline mutations [145, 146]. The variable phenotypes inherent to such experiments demands caution when drawing conclusions and requires validation in germline mutants; however, the risk of false negatives is likely greater than false positives if the concentration of Cas9 and single guide-RNA (sgRNAs) have been optimized [145]. Furthermore, by injected Cas9 protein rather than Cas9-encoding mRNA, it is possible to increase efficiency and generate biallelic mutations very early in development [146].

CONCLUDING REMARKS

Visual impairment is a common symptom of ciliopathies but the links between clinical symptoms and cilia dysfunction are not entirely clear. While photoreceptors remain the prime candidate for ciliary dysfunction, other tissues of the eye can be perturbed. Cells of the corneal endothelium have cilia [147] and corneal defects are seen in patients with immotile-cilia syndrome [148]. Altering the polarization of cilia in lens fiber cells results in abnormal lens morphology [149]. Clearly, more work is needed to understand all the causes of vision loss in these diseases.

The genetic variability in ciliopathies and the difficulty associated with accurately correlating genotype to phenotype will require much more research in animal models. The genomics infrastructure, tools for reverse genetics, and economics (*i.e.* cost per animal) continue to make zebrafish an attractive choice for genetic studies of human disease. The growing use of TALEN and CRISPR/Cas9 technology will facilitate the generation of ciliopathy mutants that can be used to verify morphant phenotypes and these technologies will also enable the creation of lines harboring specific alleles known to cause disease. These models will improve our understanding of how the mutant proteins function within photoreceptors and what causes ocular dysfunction in ciliopathies.

CONFLICT OF INTEREST

The author (editor) declares no conflict of interest, financial or otherwise.

ACKNOWLEDGEMENTS

I would like to thank Dr. James Fadool (Florida State University) for useful comments on the manuscript. This work was supported by grants from the National Institutes of Health (EY017037 and EY021865) and from a Doris and Jules Stein Professorship from Research to Prevent Blindness (RPB).

REFERENCES

[1]   Prensier G, Vivier E, Goldstein S, Schrével J. Motile flagellum with a "3 + 0" ultrastructure. Science 1980; 207(4438): 1493-4.
[http://dx.doi.org/10.1126/science.7189065] [PMID: 7189065]

[2]   Hildebrandt F, Benzing T, Katsanis N. Ciliopathies. N Engl J Med 2011; 364(16): 1533-43.
[http://dx.doi.org/10.1056/NEJMra1010172] [PMID: 21506742]

[3]   Novarino G, Akizu N, Gleeson JG. Modeling human disease in humans: the ciliopathies. Cell 2011; 147(1): 70-9.
[http://dx.doi.org/10.1016/j.cell.2011.09.014] [PMID: 21962508]

[4]   Gerdes JM, Katsanis N. Ciliary function and Wnt signal modulation. Curr Top Dev Biol 2008; 85: 175-95.
[http://dx.doi.org/10.1016/S0070-2153(08)00807-7] [PMID: 19147006]

[5]   Nozawa YI, Lin C, Chuang PT. Hedgehog signaling from the primary cilium to the nucleus: an emerging picture of ciliary localization, trafficking and transduction. Curr Opin Genet Dev 2013; 23(4): 429-37.
[http://dx.doi.org/10.1016/j.gde.2013.04.008] [PMID: 23725801]

[6]   May-Simera HL, Kelley MW. Cilia, Wnt signaling, and the cytoskeleton. Cilia 2012; 1(1): 7.
[http://dx.doi.org/10.1186/2046-2530-1-7] [PMID: 23351924]

[7]   Wallingford JB, Mitchell B. Strange as it may seem: the many links between Wnt signaling, planar cell polarity, and cilia. Genes Dev 2011; 25(3): 201-13.
[http://dx.doi.org/10.1101/gad.2008011] [PMID: 21289065]

[8]   Scholey JM, Anderson KV. Intraflagellar transport and cilium-based signaling. Cell 2006; 125(3): 439-42.
[http://dx.doi.org/10.1016/j.cell.2006.04.013] [PMID: 16678091]

[9]   Guemez-Gamboa A, Coufal NG, Gleeson JG. Primary cilia in the developing and mature brain. Neuron 2014; 82(3): 511-21.
[http://dx.doi.org/10.1016/j.neuron.2014.04.024] [PMID: 24811376]

[10]   Gerdes JM, Davis EE, Katsanis N. The vertebrate primary cilium in development, homeostasis, and disease. Cell 2009; 137(1): 32-45.
[http://dx.doi.org/10.1016/j.cell.2009.03.023] [PMID: 19345185]

[11]   Valente EM, Rosti RO, Gibbs E, Gleeson JG. Primary cilia in neurodevelopmental disorders. Nat Rev Neurol 2014; 10(1): 27-36.
[http://dx.doi.org/10.1038/nrneurol.2013.247] [PMID: 24296655]

[12]   Scholey JM. Intraflagellar transport. Annu Rev Cell Dev Biol 2003; 19: 423-43.
[http://dx.doi.org/10.1146/annurev.cellbio.19.111401.091318] [PMID: 14570576]

[13]   Scholey JM. Kinesin-2: a family of heterotrimeric and homodimeric motors with diverse intracellular transport functions. Annu Rev Cell Dev Biol 2013; 29: 443-69.
[http://dx.doi.org/10.1146/annurev-cellbio-101512-122335] [PMID: 23750925]

[14]   Malicki J, Besharse JC. Kinesin-2 family motors in the unusual photoreceptor cilium. Vision Res

2012; 75: 33-6.
[http://dx.doi.org/10.1016/j.visres.2012.10.008] [PMID: 23123805]

[15]   Carvalho-Santos Z, Azimzadeh J, Pereira-Leal JB, Bettencourt-Dias M. Evolution: Tracing the origins of centrioles, cilia, and flagella. J Cell Biol 2011; 194(2): 165-75.
[http://dx.doi.org/10.1083/jcb.201011152] [PMID: 21788366]

[16]   Sung CH, Leroux MR. The roles of evolutionarily conserved functional modules in cilia-related trafficking. Nat Cell Biol 2013; 15(12): 1387-97.
[http://dx.doi.org/10.1038/ncb2888] [PMID: 24296415]

[17]   De Robertis E. Electron microscope observations on the submicroscopic organization of the retinal rods. J Biophys Biochem Cytol 1956; 2(3): 319-30.
[http://dx.doi.org/10.1083/jcb.2.3.319] [PMID: 13331964]

[18]   Liu Q, Tan G, Levenkova N, *et al.* The proteome of the mouse photoreceptor sensory cilium complex. Mol Cell Proteomics 2007; 6(8): 1299-317.
[http://dx.doi.org/10.1074/mcp.M700054-MCP200] [PMID: 17494944]

[19]   De Robertis E. Some observations on the ultrastructure and morphogenesis of photoreceptors. J Gen Physiol 1960; 43(6) (Suppl.): 1-13.
[http://dx.doi.org/10.1085/jgp.43.6.1] [PMID: 13814989]

[20]   Besharse JC, Forestner DM, Defoe DM. Membrane assembly in retinal photoreceptors. III. Distinct membrane domains of the connecting cilium of developing rods. J Neurosci 1985; 5(4): 1035-48.
[PMID: 3156973]

[21]   Besharse JC, Pfenninger KH. Membrane assembly in retinal photoreceptors I. Freeze-fracture analysis of cytoplasmic vesicles in relationship to disc assembly. J Cell Biol 1980; 87(2 Pt 1): 451-63.
[http://dx.doi.org/10.1083/jcb.87.2.451] [PMID: 7430251]

[22]   Gilliam JC, Chang JT, Sandoval IM, *et al.* Three-dimensional architecture of the rod sensory cilium and its disruption in retinal neurodegeneration. Cell 2012; 151(5): 1029-41.
[http://dx.doi.org/10.1016/j.cell.2012.10.038] [PMID: 23178122]

[23]   Steinberg RH, Wood I. Clefts and microtubules of photoreceptor outer segments in the retina of the domestic cat. J Ultrastruct Res 1975; 51(3): 307-403.
[http://dx.doi.org/10.1016/S0022-5320(75)80102-X] [PMID: 1138108]

[24]   Insinna C, Pathak N, Perkins B, Drummond I, Besharse JC. The homodimeric kinesin, Kif17, is essential for vertebrate photoreceptor sensory outer segment development. Dev Biol 2008; 316(1): 160-70.
[http://dx.doi.org/10.1016/j.ydbio.2008.01.025] [PMID: 18304522]

[25]   Marszalek JR, Liu X, Roberts EA, *et al.* Genetic evidence for selective transport of opsin and arrestin by kinesin-II in mammalian photoreceptors. Cell 2000; 102(2): 175-87.
[http://dx.doi.org/10.1016/S0092-8674(00)00023-4] [PMID: 10943838]

[26]   Pazour GJ, Baker SA, Deane JA, *et al.* The intraflagellar transport protein, IFT88, is essential for vertebrate photoreceptor assembly and maintenance. J Cell Biol 2002; 157(1): 103-13.
[http://dx.doi.org/10.1083/jcb.200107108] [PMID: 11916979]

[27]   Tsujikawa M, Malicki J. Intraflagellar transport genes are essential for differentiation and survival of vertebrate sensory neurons. Neuron 2004; 42(5): 703-16.
[http://dx.doi.org/10.1016/S0896-6273(04)00268-5] [PMID: 15182712]

[28]   Krock BL, Mills-Henry I, Perkins BD. Retrograde intraflagellar transport by cytoplasmic dynein-2 is required for outer segment extension in vertebrate photoreceptors but not arrestin translocation. Invest Ophthalmol Vis Sci 2009; 50(11): 5463-71.
[http://dx.doi.org/10.1167/iovs.09-3828] [PMID: 19474410]

[29]   Krock BL, Perkins BD. The intraflagellar transport protein IFT57 is required for cilia maintenance and regulates IFT-particle-kinesin-II dissociation in vertebrate photoreceptors. J Cell Sci 2008; 121(11):

1907-15.
[http://dx.doi.org/10.1242/jcs.029397] [PMID: 18492793]

[30]   Insinna C, Humby M, Sedmak T, Wolfrum U, Besharse JC. Different roles for KIF17 and kinesin II in photoreceptor development and maintenance. Dev Dyn 2009; 238(9): 2211-22.
[http://dx.doi.org/10.1002/dvdy.21956] [PMID: 19384852]

[31]   Ishikawa H, Marshall WF. Ciliogenesis: building the cell's antenna. Nat Rev Mol Cell Biol 2011; 12(4): 222-34.
[http://dx.doi.org/10.1038/nrm3085] [PMID: 21427764]

[32]   Hou Y, Witman GB. Dynein and intraflagellar transport. Exp Cell Res 2015; 334(1): 26-34.
[http://dx.doi.org/10.1016/j.yexcr.2015.02.017] [PMID: 25725253]

[33]   Insinna C, Besharse JC. Intraflagellar transport and the sensory outer segment of vertebrate photoreceptors. Dev Dyn 2008; 237(8): 1982-92.
[http://dx.doi.org/10.1002/dvdy.21554] [PMID: 18489002]

[34]   Liu Q, Zhang Q, Pierce EA. Photoreceptor sensory cilia and inherited retinal degeneration. Adv Exp Med Biol 2010; 664: 223-32.
[http://dx.doi.org/10.1007/978-1-4419-1399-9_26] [PMID: 20238021]

[35]   Sahly I, Dufour E, Schietroma C, *et al.* Localization of Usher 1 proteins to the photoreceptor calyceal processes, which are absent from mice. J Cell Biol 2012; 199(2): 381-99.
[http://dx.doi.org/10.1083/jcb.201202012] [PMID: 23045546]

[36]   Brown PK, Gibbons IR, Wald G. The visual cells and visual pigment of the mudpuppy, necturus. J Cell Biol 1963; 19: 79-106.
[http://dx.doi.org/10.1083/jcb.19.1.79] [PMID: 14069804]

[37]   Branchek T, Bremiller R. The development of photoreceptors in the zebrafish, Brachydanio rerio. I. Structure. J Comp Neurol 1984; 224(1): 107-15.
[http://dx.doi.org/10.1002/cne.902240109] [PMID: 6715574]

[38]   Raymond PA, Barthel LK, Rounsifer ME, Sullivan SA, Knight JK. Expression of rod and cone visual pigments in goldfish and zebrafish: a rhodopsin-like gene is expressed in cones. Neuron 1993; 10(6): 1161-74.
[http://dx.doi.org/10.1016/0896-6273(93)90064-X] [PMID: 8318234]

[39]   Ramsey M, Perkins BD. Basal bodies exhibit polarized positioning in zebrafish cone photoreceptors. J Comp Neurol 2013; 521(8): 1803-16.
[http://dx.doi.org/10.1002/cne.23260] [PMID: 23171982]

[40]   Knabe W, Kuhn HJ. Ciliogenesis in photoreceptor cells of the tree shrew retina. Anat Embryol (Berl) 1997; 196(2): 123-31.
[http://dx.doi.org/10.1007/s004290050085] [PMID: 9278157]

[41]   Badano JL, Mitsuma N, Beales PL, Katsanis N. The ciliopathies: an emerging class of human genetic disorders. Annu Rev Genomics Hum Genet 2006; 7: 125-48.
[http://dx.doi.org/10.1146/annurev.genom.7.080505.115610] [PMID: 16722803]

[42]   Kartagener M. Zur pathogenese der bronchiektasien: bronchiektasien bei situs viscerum inversus. Bielt Kin Tuberk 1933; 83: 489-501.
[http://dx.doi.org/10.1007/BF02141468]

[43]   Vague J, Farnarier G, Sobrepere G. Laurence-Moon-Bardet-Biedl syndrome. Rev Otoneuroophtalmol 1950; 22(1): 60-3.
[PMID: 15424572]

[44]   Joubert M, Eisenring JJ, Andermann F. Familial dysgenesis of the vermis: a syndrome of hyperventilation, abnormal eye movements and retardation. Neurology 1968; 18(3): 302-3.
[PMID: 5690407]

[45]   Afzelius BA. A human syndrome caused by immotile cilia. Science 1976; 193(4250): 317-9.
       [http://dx.doi.org/10.1126/science.1084576] [PMID: 1084576]

[46]   Kozminski KG, Beech PL, Rosenbaum JL. The Chlamydomonas kinesin-like protein FLA10 is
       involved in motility associated with the flagellar membrane. J Cell Biol 1995; 131(6 Pt 1): 1517-27.
       [http://dx.doi.org/10.1083/jcb.131.6.1517] [PMID: 8522608]

[47]   Kozminski KG, Johnson KA, Forscher P, Rosenbaum JL. A motility in the eukaryotic flagellum
       unrelated to flagellar beating. Proc Natl Acad Sci USA 1993; 90(12): 5519-23.
       [http://dx.doi.org/10.1073/pnas.90.12.5519] [PMID: 8516294]

[48]   Cole DG, Diener DR, Himelblau AL, Beech PL, Fuster JC, Rosenbaum JL. Chlamydomonas kinesin-
       II-dependent intraflagellar transport (IFT): IFT particles contain proteins required for ciliary assembly
       in Caenorhabditis elegans sensory neurons. J Cell Biol 1998; 141(4): 993-1008.
       [http://dx.doi.org/10.1083/jcb.141.4.993] [PMID: 9585417]

[49]   Pazour GJ, Dickert BL, Witman GB. The DHC1b (DHC2) isoform of cytoplasmic dynein is required
       for flagellar assembly. J Cell Biol 1999; 144(3): 473-81.
       [http://dx.doi.org/10.1083/jcb.144.3.473] [PMID: 9971742]

[50]   Pazour GJ, Wilkerson CG, Witman GB. A dynein light chain is essential for the retrograde particle
       movement of intraflagellar transport (IFT). J Cell Biol 1998; 141(4): 979-92.
       [http://dx.doi.org/10.1083/jcb.141.4.979] [PMID: 9585416]

[51]   Perkins LA, Hedgecock EM, Thomson JN, Culotti JG. Mutant sensory cilia in the nematode
       Caenorhabditis elegans. Dev Biol 1986; 117(2): 456-87.
       [http://dx.doi.org/10.1016/0012-1606(86)90314-3] [PMID: 2428682]

[52]   Signor D, Wedaman KP, Orozco JT, *et al.* Role of a class DHC1b dynein in retrograde transport of
       IFT motors and IFT raft particles along cilia, but not dendrites, in chemosensory neurons of living
       Caenorhabditis elegans. J Cell Biol 1999; 147(3): 519-30.
       [http://dx.doi.org/10.1083/jcb.147.3.519] [PMID: 10545497]

[53]   Doerre G, Malicki J. Genetic analysis of photoreceptor cell development in the zebrafish retina. Mech
       Dev 2002; 110(1-2): 125-38.
       [http://dx.doi.org/10.1016/S0925-4773(01)00571-8] [PMID: 11744374]

[54]   Schrick JJ, Onuchic LF, Reeders ST, *et al.* Characterization of the human homologue of the mouse
       Tg737 candidate polycystic kidney disease gene. Hum Mol Genet 1995; 4(4): 559-67.
       [http://dx.doi.org/10.1093/hmg/4.4.559] [PMID: 7633404]

[55]   Yoder BK, Richards WG, Sweeney WE, Wilkinson JE, Avener ED, Woychik RP. Insertional
       mutagenesis and molecular analysis of a new gene associated with polycystic kidney disease. Proc
       Assoc Am Physicians 1995; 107(3): 314-23.
       [PMID: 8608416]

[56]   Yoder BK, Tousson A, Millican L, *et al.* Polaris, a protein disrupted in orpk mutant mice, is required
       for assembly of renal cilium. Am J Physiol Renal Physiol 2002; 282(3): F541-52.
       [http://dx.doi.org/10.1152/ajprenal.00273.2001] [PMID: 11832437]

[57]   Haycraft CJ, Swoboda P, Taulman PD, Thomas JH, Yoder BK. The C. elegans homolog of the murine
       cystic kidney disease gene Tg737 functions in a ciliogenic pathway and is disrupted in osm-5 mutant
       worms. Development 2001; 128(9): 1493-505.
       [PMID: 11290289]

[58]   Denniston AK, Beales PL, Tomlins PJ, *et al.* Evaluation of visual function and needs in adult patients
       with bardet-biedl syndrome. Retina 2014; 34(11): 2282-9.
       [http://dx.doi.org/10.1097/IAE.0000000000000222] [PMID: 25170860]

[59]   Mockel A, Perdomo Y, Stutzmann F, Letsch J, Marion V, Dollfus H. Retinal dystrophy in Bardet-
       Biedl syndrome and related syndromic ciliopathies. Prog Retin Eye Res 2011; 30(4): 258-74.
       [http://dx.doi.org/10.1016/j.preteyeres.2011.03.001] [PMID: 21477661]

[60]   Ansley SJ, Badano JL, Blacque OE, *et al.* Basal body dysfunction is a likely cause of pleiotropic Bardet-Biedl syndrome. Nature 2003; 425(6958): 628-33.
[http://dx.doi.org/10.1038/nature02030] [PMID: 14520415]

[61]   Khan AO, Oystreck DT, Seidahmed MZ, *et al.* Ophthalmic features of Joubert syndrome. Ophthalmology 2008; 115(12): 2286-9.
[http://dx.doi.org/10.1016/j.ophtha.2008.08.005] [PMID: 19041481]

[62]   Maria BL, Boltshauser E, Palmer SC, Tran TX. Clinical features and revised diagnostic criteria in Joubert syndrome. J Child Neurol 1999; 14(9): 583-90.
[http://dx.doi.org/10.1177/088307389901400906] [PMID: 10488903]

[63]   Steinlin M, Schmid M, Landau K, Boltshauser E. Follow-up in children with Joubert syndrome. Neuropediatrics 1997; 28(4): 204-11.
[http://dx.doi.org/10.1055/s-2007-973701] [PMID: 9309710]

[64]   Cantagrel V, Silhavy JL, Bielas SL, *et al.* Mutations in the cilia gene ARL13B lead to the classical form of Joubert syndrome. Am J Hum Genet 2008; 83(2): 170-9.
[http://dx.doi.org/10.1016/j.ajhg.2008.06.023] [PMID: 18674751]

[65]   Roepman R, Letteboer SJ, Arts HH, *et al.* Interaction of nephrocystin-4 and RPGRIP1 is disrupted by nephronophthisis or Leber congenital amaurosis-associated mutations. Proc Natl Acad Sci USA 2005; 102(51): 18520-5.
[http://dx.doi.org/10.1073/pnas.0505774102] [PMID: 16339905]

[66]   Casteels I, Demandt E, Legius E. Visual loss as the presenting sign of Jeune syndrome. Eur J Paediatr Neurol 2000; 4(5): 243-7.
[http://dx.doi.org/10.1053/ejpn.2000.0313] [PMID: 11030072]

[67]   Khanna H, Davis EE, Murga-Zamalloa CA, *et al.* A common allele in RPGRIP1L is a modifier of retinal degeneration in ciliopathies. Nat Genet 2009; 41(6): 739-45.
[http://dx.doi.org/10.1038/ng.366] [PMID: 19430481]

[68]   Katsanis N. The oligogenic properties of Bardet-Biedl syndrome. Hum Mol Genet 2004; 13(Spec No 1): R65-71.
[http://dx.doi.org/10.1093/hmg/ddh092] [PMID: 14976158]

[69]   Haffter P, Granato M, Brand M, *et al.* The identification of genes with unique and essential functions in the development of the zebrafish, Danio rerio. Development 1996; 123: 1-36.
[PMID: 9007226]

[70]   Driever W, Solnica-Krezel L, Schier AF, *et al.* A genetic screen for mutations affecting embryogenesis in zebrafish. Development 1996; 123: 37-46.
[PMID: 9007227]

[71]   Malicki J, Neuhauss SC, Schier AF, *et al.* Mutations affecting development of the zebrafish retina. Development 1996; 123: 263-73.
[PMID: 9007246]

[72]   Drummond IA, Majumdar A, Hentschel H, *et al.* Early development of the zebrafish pronephros and analysis of mutations affecting pronephric function. Development 1998; 125(23): 4655-67.
[PMID: 9806915]

[73]   Sun Z, Amsterdam A, Pazour GJ, Cole DG, Miller MS, Hopkins N. A genetic screen in zebrafish identifies cilia genes as a principal cause of cystic kidney. Development 2004; 131(16): 4085-93.
[http://dx.doi.org/10.1242/dev.01240] [PMID: 15269167]

[74]   Gross JM, Perkins BD. Zebrafish mutants as models for congenital ocular disorders in humans. Mol Reprod Dev 2008; 75(3): 547-55.
[http://dx.doi.org/10.1002/mrd.20831] [PMID: 18058918]

[75]   Ryan S, Willer J, Marjoram L, *et al.* Rapid identification of kidney cyst mutations by whole exome

sequencing in zebrafish. Development 2013; 140(21): 4445-51.
[http://dx.doi.org/10.1242/dev.101170] [PMID: 24130329]

[76]   Pathak N, Obara T, Mangos S, Liu Y, Drummond IA. The zebrafish fleer gene encodes an essential
       regulator of cilia tubulin polyglutamylation. Mol Biol Cell 2007; 18(11): 4353-64.
       [http://dx.doi.org/10.1091/mbc.E07-06-0537] [PMID: 17761526]

[77]   Bachmann-Gagescu R, Phelps IG, Stearns G, *et al.* The ciliopathy gene cc2d2a controls zebrafish
       photoreceptor outer segment development through a role in Rab8-dependent vesicle trafficking. Hum
       Mol Genet 2011; 20(20): 4041-55.
       [http://dx.doi.org/10.1093/hmg/ddr332] [PMID: 21816947]

[78]   Otto EA, Schermer B, Obara T, *et al.* Mutations in INVS encoding inversin cause nephronophthisis
       type 2, linking renal cystic disease to the function of primary cilia and left-right axis determination.
       Nat Genet 2003; 34(4): 413-20.
       [http://dx.doi.org/10.1038/ng1217] [PMID: 12872123]

[79]   Hudak LM, Lunt S, Chang CH, *et al.* The intraflagellar transport protein ift80 is essential for
       photoreceptor survival in a zebrafish model of jeune asphyxiating thoracic dystrophy. Invest
       Ophthalmol Vis Sci 2010; 51(7): 3792-9.
       [http://dx.doi.org/10.1167/iovs.09-4312] [PMID: 20207966]

[80]   Zaghloul NA, Liu Y, Gerdes JM, *et al.* Functional analyses of variants reveal a significant role for
       dominant negative and common alleles in oligogenic Bardet-Biedl syndrome. Proc Natl Acad Sci USA
       2010; 107(23): 10602-7.
       [http://dx.doi.org/10.1073/pnas.1000219107] [PMID: 20498079]

[81]   Ross AJ, May-Simera H, Eichers ER, *et al.* Disruption of Bardet-Biedl syndrome ciliary proteins
       perturbs planar cell polarity in vertebrates. Nat Genet 2005; 37(10): 1135-40.
       [http://dx.doi.org/10.1038/ng1644] [PMID: 16170314]

[82]   Yen HJ, Tayeh MK, Mullins RF, Stone EM, Sheffield VC, Slusarski DC. Bardet-Biedl syndrome
       genes are important in retrograde intracellular trafficking and Kupffer's vesicle cilia function. Hum
       Mol Genet 2006; 15(5): 667-77.
       [http://dx.doi.org/10.1093/hmg/ddi468] [PMID: 16399798]

[83]   Sayer JA, Otto EA, O'Toole JF, *et al.* The centrosomal protein nephrocystin-6 is mutated in Joubert
       syndrome and activates transcription factor ATF4. Nat Genet 2006; 38(6): 674-81.
       [http://dx.doi.org/10.1038/ng1786] [PMID: 16682973]

[84]   Murga-Zamalloa CA, Ghosh AK, Patil SB, *et al.* Accumulation of the Raf-1 kinase inhibitory protein
       (Rkip) is associated with Cep290-mediated photoreceptor degeneration in ciliopathies. J Biol Chem
       2011; 286(32): 28276-86.
       [http://dx.doi.org/10.1074/jbc.M111.237560] [PMID: 21685394]

[85]   Veleri S, Bishop K, Dalle Nogare DE, *et al.* Knockdown of Bardet-Biedl syndrome gene
       BBS9/PTHB1 leads to cilia defects. PLoS One 2012; 7(3): e34389.
       [http://dx.doi.org/10.1371/journal.pone.0034389] [PMID: 22479622]

[86]   Ghosh AK, Murga-Zamalloa CA, Chan L, Hitchcock PF, Swaroop A, Khanna H. Human retinopathy-
       associated ciliary protein retinitis pigmentosa GTPase regulator mediates cilia-dependent vertebrate
       development. Hum Mol Genet 2010; 19(1): 90-8.
       [http://dx.doi.org/10.1093/hmg/ddp469] [PMID: 19815619]

[87]   Seo S, Baye LM, Schulz NP, *et al.* BBS6, BBS10, and BBS12 form a complex with CCT/TRiC family
       chaperonins and mediate BBSome assembly. Proc Natl Acad Sci USA 2010; 107(4): 1488-93.
       [http://dx.doi.org/10.1073/pnas.0910268107] [PMID: 20080638]

[88]   Valente EM, Logan CV, Mougou-Zerelli S, *et al.* Mutations in TMEM216 perturb ciliogenesis and
       cause Joubert, Meckel and related syndromes. Nat Genet 2010; 42(7): 619-25.
       [http://dx.doi.org/10.1038/ng.594] [PMID: 20512146]

[89] Huang L, Szymanska K, Jensen VL, *et al.* TMEM237 is mutated in individuals with a Joubert syndrome related disorder and expands the role of the TMEM family at the ciliary transition zone. Am J Hum Genet 2011; 89(6): 713-30.
[http://dx.doi.org/10.1016/j.ajhg.2011.11.005] [PMID: 22152675]

[90] Lee JE, Silhavy JL, Zaki MS, *et al.* CEP41 is mutated in Joubert syndrome and is required for tubulin glutamylation at the cilium. Nat Genet 2012; 44(2): 193-9.
[http://dx.doi.org/10.1038/ng.1078] [PMID: 22246503]

[91] Mitchison HM, Schmidts M, Loges NT, Freshour J, Dritsoula A, Hirst RA, *et al.* Mutations in axonemal dynein assembly factor DNAAF3 cause primary ciliary dyskinesia. Nat Genet 2012; 44(4): 381-9.
[http://dx.doi.org/10.1038/ng.1106]

[92] Gross JM, Perkins BD, Amsterdam A, *et al.* Identification of zebrafish insertional mutants with defects in visual system development and function. Genetics 2005; 170(1): 245-61.
[http://dx.doi.org/10.1534/genetics.104.039727] [PMID: 15716491]

[93] Sukumaran S, Perkins BD. Early defects in photoreceptor outer segment morphogenesis in zebrafish ift57, ift88 and ift172 Intraflagellar Transport mutants. Vision Res 2009; 49(4): 479-89.
[http://dx.doi.org/10.1016/j.visres.2008.12.009] [PMID: 19136023]

[94] Moyer JH, Lee-Tischler MJ, Kwon HY, *et al.* Candidate gene associated with a mutation causing recessive polycystic kidney disease in mice. Science 1994; 264(5163): 1329-33.
[http://dx.doi.org/10.1126/science.8191288] [PMID: 8191288]

[95] Zaghloul NA, Katsanis N. Mechanistic insights into Bardet-Biedl syndrome, a model ciliopathy. J Clin Invest 2009; 119(3): 428-37.
[http://dx.doi.org/10.1172/JCI37041] [PMID: 19252258]

[96] Fan Y, Esmail MA, Ansley SJ, *et al.* Mutations in a member of the Ras superfamily of small GTP-binding proteins causes Bardet-Biedl syndrome. Nat Genet 2004; 36(9): 989-93.
[http://dx.doi.org/10.1038/ng1414] [PMID: 15314642]

[97] Riazuddin SA, Zaghloul NA, Al-Saif A, *et al.* Missense mutations in TCF8 cause late-onset Fuchs corneal dystrophy and interact with FCD4 on chromosome 9p. Am J Hum Genet 2010; 86(1): 45-53.
[http://dx.doi.org/10.1016/j.ajhg.2009.12.001] [PMID: 20036349]

[98] Pawlik B, Mir A, Iqbal H, *et al.* A novel familial bbs12 mutation associated with a mild phenotype: implications for clinical and molecular diagnostic strategies. Mol Syndromol 2010; 1(1): 27-34.
[http://dx.doi.org/10.1159/000276763] [PMID: 20648243]

[99] Estrada-Cuzcano A, Koenekoop RK, Senechal A, *et al.* BBS1 mutations in a wide spectrum of phenotypes ranging from nonsyndromic retinitis pigmentosa to Bardet-Biedl syndrome. Arch Ophthalmol 2012; 130(11): 1425-32.
[http://dx.doi.org/10.1001/archophthalmol.2012.2434] [PMID: 23143442]

[100] Shevach E, Ali M, Mizrahi-Meissonnier L, *et al.* Association between missense mutations in the BBS2 gene and nonsyndromic retinitis pigmentosa. JAMA Ophthalmol 2015; 133(3): 312-8.
[http://dx.doi.org/10.1001/jamaophthalmol.2014.5251] [PMID: 25541840]

[101] Stoetzel C, Laurier V, Davis EE, *et al.* BBS10 encodes a vertebrate-specific chaperonin-like protein and is a major BBS locus. Nat Genet 2006; 38(5): 521-4.
[http://dx.doi.org/10.1038/ng1771] [PMID: 16582908]

[102] Stoetzel C, Muller J, Laurier V, *et al.* Identification of a novel BBS gene (BBS12) highlights the major role of a vertebrate-specific branch of chaperonin-related proteins in Bardet-Biedl syndrome. Am J Hum Genet 2007; 80(1): 1-11.
[http://dx.doi.org/10.1086/510256] [PMID: 17160889]

[103] Leitch CC, Zaghloul NA, Davis EE, *et al.* Hypomorphic mutations in syndromic encephalocele genes are associated with Bardet-Biedl syndrome. Nat Genet 2008; 40(4): 443-8.

[http://dx.doi.org/10.1038/ng.97] [PMID: 18327255]

[104] Gerdes JM, Liu Y, Zaghloul NA, *et al.* Disruption of the basal body compromises proteasomal function and perturbs intracellular Wnt response. Nat Genet 2007; 39(11): 1350-60.
       [http://dx.doi.org/10.1038/ng.2007.12] [PMID: 17906624]

[105] Badano JL, Kim JC, Hoskins BE, *et al.* Heterozygous mutations in BBS1, BBS2 and BBS6 have a potential epistatic effect on Bardet-Biedl patients with two mutations at a second BBS locus. Hum Mol Genet 2003; 12(14): 1651-9.
       [http://dx.doi.org/10.1093/hmg/ddg188] [PMID: 12837689]

[106] Loktev AV, Zhang Q, Beck JS, *et al.* A BBSome subunit links ciliogenesis, microtubule stability, and acetylation. Dev Cell 2008; 15(6): 854-65.
       [http://dx.doi.org/10.1016/j.devcel.2008.11.001] [PMID: 19081074]

[107] Borovina A, Ciruna B. IFT88 plays a cilia- and PCP-independent role in controlling oriented cell divisions during vertebrate embryonic development. Cell Reports 2013; 5(1): 37-43.
       [http://dx.doi.org/10.1016/j.celrep.2013.08.043] [PMID: 24095732]

[108] Pretorius PR, Baye LM, Nishimura DY, *et al.* Identification and functional analysis of the vision-specific BBS3 (ARL6) long isoform. PLoS Genet 2010; 6(3): e1000884.
       [http://dx.doi.org/10.1371/journal.pgen.1000884] [PMID: 20333246]

[109] Wang H, Chen X, Dudinsky L, *et al.* Exome capture sequencing identifies a novel mutation in BBS4. Mol Vis 2011; 17: 3529-40.
       [PMID: 22219648]

[110] Chamling X, Seo S, Searby CC, Kim G, Slusarski DC, Sheffield VC. The centriolar satellite protein AZI1 interacts with BBS4 and regulates ciliary trafficking of the BBSome. PLoS Genet 2014; 10(2): e1004083.
       [http://dx.doi.org/10.1371/journal.pgen.1004083] [PMID: 24550735]

[111] Zaghloul NA, Katsanis N. Zebrafish assays of ciliopathies. Methods Cell Biol 2011; 105: 257-72.
       [http://dx.doi.org/10.1016/B978-0-12-381320-6.00011-4] [PMID: 21951534]

[112] Wallingford JB, Fraser SE, Harland RM. Convergent extension: the molecular control of polarized cell movement during embryonic development. Dev Cell 2002; 2(6): 695-706.
       [http://dx.doi.org/10.1016/S1534-5807(02)00197-1] [PMID: 12062082]

[113] Wallingford JB, Rowning BA, Vogeli KM, Rothbächer U, Fraser SE, Harland RM. Dishevelled controls cell polarity during Xenopus gastrulation. Nature 2000; 405(6782): 81-5.
       [http://dx.doi.org/10.1038/35011077] [PMID: 10811222]

[114] Heisenberg CP, Tada M, Rauch GJ, *et al.* Silberblick/Wnt11 mediates convergent extension movements during zebrafish gastrulation. Nature 2000; 405(6782): 76-81.
       [http://dx.doi.org/10.1038/35011068] [PMID: 10811221]

[115] Park TJ, Mitchell BJ, Abitua PB, Kintner C, Wallingford JB. Dishevelled controls apical docking and planar polarization of basal bodies in ciliated epithelial cells. Nat Genet 2008; 40(7): 871-9.
       [http://dx.doi.org/10.1038/ng.104] [PMID: 18552847]

[116] Mitchell B, Stubbs JL, Huisman F, Taborek P, Yu C, Kintner C. The PCP pathway instructs the planar orientation of ciliated cells in the Xenopus larval skin. Curr Biol 2009; 19(11): 924-9.
       [http://dx.doi.org/10.1016/j.cub.2009.04.018] [PMID: 19427216]

[117] May-Simera HL, Kai M, Hernandez V, Osborn DP, Tada M, Beales PL. Bbs8, together with the planar cell polarity protein Vangl2, is required to establish left-right asymmetry in zebrafish. Dev Biol 2010; 345(2): 215-25.
       [http://dx.doi.org/10.1016/j.ydbio.2010.07.013] [PMID: 20643117]

[118] Jones C, Roper VC, Foucher I, *et al.* Ciliary proteins link basal body polarization to planar cell polarity regulation. Nat Genet 2008; 40(1): 69-77.
       [http://dx.doi.org/10.1038/ng.2007.54] [PMID: 18066062]

[119] Borovina A, Superina S, Voskas D, Ciruna B. Vangl2 directs the posterior tilting and asymmetric localization of motile primary cilia. Nat Cell Biol 2010; 12(4): 407-12.
[http://dx.doi.org/10.1038/ncb2042] [PMID: 20305649]

[120] Park TJ, Haigo SL, Wallingford JB. Ciliogenesis defects in embryos lacking inturned or fuzzy function are associated with failure of planar cell polarity and Hedgehog signaling. Nat Genet 2006; 38(3): 303-11.
[http://dx.doi.org/10.1038/ng1753] [PMID: 16493421]

[121] Fischer E, Legue E, Doyen A, *et al.* Defective planar cell polarity in polycystic kidney disease. Nat Genet 2006; 38(1): 21-3.
[http://dx.doi.org/10.1038/ng1701] [PMID: 16341222]

[122] Oh EC, Katsanis N. Cilia in vertebrate development and disease. Development 2012; 139(3): 443-8.
[http://dx.doi.org/10.1242/dev.050054] [PMID: 22223675]

[123] Oh EC, Katsanis N. Context-dependent regulation of Wnt signaling through the primary cilium. J Am Soc Nephrol 2013; 24(1): 10-8.
[http://dx.doi.org/10.1681/ASN.2012050526] [PMID: 23123400]

[124] Sattar S, Gleeson JG. The ciliopathies in neuronal development: a clinical approach to investigation of Joubert syndrome and Joubert syndrome-related disorders. Dev Med Child Neurol 2011; 53(9): 793-8.
[http://dx.doi.org/10.1111/j.1469-8749.2011.04021.x] [PMID: 21679365]

[125] Thomas S, Wright KJ, Le Corre S, *et al.* A homozygous PDE6D mutation in Joubert syndrome impairs targeting of farnesylated INPP5E protein to the primary cilium. Hum Mutat 2014; 35(1): 137-46.
[http://dx.doi.org/10.1002/humu.22470] [PMID: 24166846]

[126] Tuz K, Bachmann-Gagescu R, O'Day DR, *et al.* Mutations in CSPP1 cause primary cilia abnormalities and Joubert syndrome with or without Jeune asphyxiating thoracic dystrophy. Am J Hum Genet 2014; 94(1): 62-72.
[http://dx.doi.org/10.1016/j.ajhg.2013.11.019] [PMID: 24360808]

[127] Davis EE, Zhang Q, Liu Q, *et al.* TTC21B contributes both causal and modifying alleles across the ciliopathy spectrum. Nat Genet 2011; 43(3): 189-96.
[http://dx.doi.org/10.1038/ng.756] [PMID: 21258341]

[128] Lindstrand A, Davis EE, Carvalho CM, *et al.* Recurrent CNVs and SNVs at the NPHP1 locus contribute pathogenic alleles to Bardet-Biedl syndrome. Am J Hum Genet 2014; 94(5): 745-54.
[http://dx.doi.org/10.1016/j.ajhg.2014.03.017] [PMID: 24746959]

[129] Simms RJ, Hynes AM, Eley L, *et al.* Modelling a ciliopathy: Ahi1 knockdown in model systems reveals an essential role in brain, retinal, and renal development. Cell Mol Life Sci 2012; 69(6): 993-1009.
[http://dx.doi.org/10.1007/s00018-011-0826-z] [PMID: 21959375]

[130] Owens KN, Santos F, Roberts B, *et al.* Identification of genetic and chemical modulators of zebrafish mechanosensory hair cell death. PLoS Genet 2008; 4(2): e1000020.
[http://dx.doi.org/10.1371/journal.pgen.1000020] [PMID: 18454195]

[131] Gorden NT, Arts HH, Parisi MA, *et al.* CC2D2A is mutated in Joubert syndrome and interacts with the ciliopathy-associated basal body protein CEP290. Am J Hum Genet 2008; 83(5): 559-71.
[http://dx.doi.org/10.1016/j.ajhg.2008.10.002] [PMID: 18950740]

[132] Chih B, Liu P, Chinn Y, *et al.* A ciliopathy complex at the transition zone protects the cilia as a privileged membrane domain. Nat Cell Biol 2011; 14(1): 61-72.
[http://dx.doi.org/10.1038/ncb2410] [PMID: 22179047]

[133] Golling G, Amsterdam A, Sun Z, *et al.* Insertional mutagenesis in zebrafish rapidly identifies genes essential for early vertebrate development. Nat Genet 2002; 31(2): 135-40.
[http://dx.doi.org/10.1038/ng896] [PMID: 12006978]

[134] Duldulao NA, Lee S, Sun Z. Cilia localization is essential for *in vivo* functions of the Joubert syndrome protein Arl13b/Scorpion. Development 2009; 136(23): 4033-42.
[http://dx.doi.org/10.1242/dev.036350] [PMID: 19906870]

[135] Thomas TJ, Seibold JR, Adams LE, Hess EV. Triplex-DNA stabilization by hydralazine and the presence of anti-(triplex DNA) antibodies in patients treated with hydralazine. Biochem J 1995; 311(Pt 1): 183-8.
[http://dx.doi.org/10.1042/bj3110183] [PMID: 7575452]

[136] Nasevicius A, Ekker SC. Effective targeted gene 'knockdown' in zebrafish. Nat Genet 2000; 26(2): 216-20.
[http://dx.doi.org/10.1038/79951] [PMID: 11017081]

[137] Fadool JM, Brockerhoff SE, Hyatt GA, Dowling JE. Mutations affecting eye morphology in the developing zebrafish (Danio rerio). Dev Genet 1997; 20(3): 288-95.
[http://dx.doi.org/10.1002/(SICI)1520-6408(1997)20:3<288::AID-DVG11>3.0.CO;2-4]   [PMID: 9216068]

[138] Muto A, Orger MB, Wehman AM, *et al.* Forward genetic analysis of visual behavior in zebrafish. PLoS Genet 2005; 1(5): e66.
[http://dx.doi.org/10.1371/journal.pgen.0010066] [PMID: 16311625]

[139] Eisen JS, Smith JC. Controlling morpholino experiments: don't stop making antisense. Development 2008; 135(10): 1735-43.
[http://dx.doi.org/10.1242/dev.001115] [PMID: 18403413]

[140] Kok FO, Shin M, Ni CW, *et al.* Reverse genetic screening reveals poor correlation between morpholino-induced and mutant phenotypes in zebrafish. Dev Cell 2015; 32(1): 97-108.
[http://dx.doi.org/10.1016/j.devcel.2014.11.018] [PMID: 25533206]

[141] Bedell VM, Wang Y, Campbell JM, *et al. In vivo* genome editing using a high-efficiency TALEN system. Nature 2012; 491(7422): 114-8.
[http://dx.doi.org/10.1038/nature11537] [PMID: 23000899]

[142] Cade L, Reyon D, Hwang WY, *et al.* Highly efficient generation of heritable zebrafish gene mutations using homo- and heterodimeric TALENs. Nucleic Acids Res 2012; 40(16): 8001-10.
[http://dx.doi.org/10.1093/nar/gks518] [PMID: 22684503]

[143] Hwang WY, Fu Y, Reyon D, *et al.* Heritable and precise zebrafish genome editing using a CRISPR-Cas system. PLoS One 2013; 8(7): e68708.
[http://dx.doi.org/10.1371/journal.pone.0068708] [PMID: 23874735]

[144] Hwang WY, Fu Y, Reyon D, *et al.* Efficient genome editing in zebrafish using a CRISPR-Cas system. Nat Biotechnol 2013; 31(3): 227-9.
[http://dx.doi.org/10.1038/nbt.2501] [PMID: 23360964]

[145] Shah AN, Davey CF, Whitebirch AC, Miller AC, Moens CB. Rapid reverse genetic screening using CRISPR in zebrafish. Nat Methods 2015; 12(6): 535-40.
[http://dx.doi.org/10.1038/nmeth.3360] [PMID: 25867848]

[146] Jao LE, Wente SR, Chen W. Efficient multiplex biallelic zebrafish genome editing using a CRISPR nuclease system. Proc Natl Acad Sci USA 2013; 110(34): 13904-9.
[http://dx.doi.org/10.1073/pnas.1308335110] [PMID: 23918387]

[147] Gallagher BC. Primary cilia of the corneal endothelium. Am J Anat 1980; 159(4): 475-84.
[http://dx.doi.org/10.1002/aja.1001590410] [PMID: 7223676]

[148] Svedbergh B, Jonsson V, Afzelius B. Immotile-cilia syndrome and the cilia of the eye. Albrecht Von Graefes Arch Klin Exp Ophthalmol 1981; 215(4): 265-72.
[http://dx.doi.org/10.1007/BF00407665] [PMID: 6971584]

[149] Sugiyama Y, Stump RJ, Nguyen A, *et al.* Secreted frizzled-related protein disrupts PCP in eye lens

fiber cells that have polarised primary cilia. Dev Biol 2010; 338(2): 193-201. [http://dx.doi.org/10.1016/j.ydbio.2009.11.033] [PMID: 19968984]

CHAPTER 3

Inositol Phosphatases in Retinal Ciliary Disorder

Cathleen Wallmuth, **Na Luo** and **Yang Sun**[*]

Indiana University School of Medicine, 1160 W. Michigan St., Indianapolis, IN 46202, USA

Abstract: Phosphoinositides are phospholipids that regulate signal transduction, endocytosis, and protein trafficking. Each phosphoinositide has a unique pattern of distribution within cellular compartments and is tightly regulated by inositol kinases and phosphatases localized within a specific membrane compartment. Inositol polyphosphate 5-phosphatases regulate phosphoinositide levels and are implicated in human diseases, such as Lowe syndrome and Joubert syndrome. Here we review the pertinent findings of the roles of 5-phosphatases in cilia function and signaling.

Keywords: Cilia, INPP5E, Joubert syndrome, Lowe syndrome, OCRL.

INTRODUCTION

Cilia are evolutionarily conserved hair-like organelles protruding from the plasma membrane (PM) of nearly all post-mitotic vertebrate cells [1 - 3]. A cilium is comprised of a nucleating basal body and a phospholipid membrane-bound axoneme that grows from the basal body during nutrition deprivation. The axoneme can be subdivided into a transition zone, axonemal stalk and a distal ciliary tip. The cilium is conventionally classified into two main types: motile and immotile/primary cilium. In the motile cilia, the outer nine sets of microtubules surround a central inner microtubule pair ("9+2" arrangement), whereas primary cilia lack the central microtubule doublet ("9+0" arrangement) [4]. This review will focus on the primary cilia.

Cilium formation (ciliogenesis) occurs in several stages. Typically it is induced when nutrition is deprived and the cell stops cell division during G1 phase of cell cycle. The mother centriole differentiates into the basal body, which associates with membrane vesicles and migrates to the cell surface where it forms the base of the primary cilium [5]. Next, elongation of the axoneme from the basal body is mediated by the transport of ciliary building proteins, a process called intraflag-

---

[*] **Corresponding author Yang Sun:** Glick Eye Institute, Department of Ophthalmology, Indiana University School of Medicine, 1160 W. Michigan Street, Indianapolis, IN 46202, United States; Tel: 301-204-1373; E-mail: sunyo@iupui.edu

ellar transport (IFT). Extension of the primary cilium occurs exclusively at the distal tip of the axoneme. Typically, there is only one primary cilium per quiescent cell; however, some cell types can develop a group of primary cilia (*e.g.* choroid plexus of the brain) [6].

Being a sensory organelle, the primary cilium plays a crucial role in embryonic development and adult tissue homeostasis [7]. Upon chemical and mechanical stimulation, the primary cilia can sense changes in the extracellular environment and initiate multiple intracellular signal transduction pathways. Hedgehog (Hhg), Wnt and platelet-derived growth factor (PDGF) signaling pathways are three typical signal transduction pathways with components localized to the primary cilia [8 - 10]. Hhg signaling pathway and its proteins specify tissue patterning in embryonic development and play an important role in post-natal homeostasis [11]. Upon binding to its receptor, the twelve-transmembrane protein Patched (Ptch), Hhg facilitates the activation of Smoothened (Smo), which in turn causes the accumulation of the active form of the transcription factor Gli in the primary cilium [12 - 14]. The disruptions of the Hhg pathway by mutations in genes that regulate ciliogenesis result in developmental disorders.

In the eyes, photoreceptors are a unique type of ciliated cells that specialize in visual phototransduction. The connecting cilium within each photoreceptor is required for the formation of the outer segment in the retina, where photosensory G protein-coupled receptor rhodopsin molecules are densely packed to allow detection of single photons [15]. The cilium is now recognized as a critical structure within the photoreceptors that mediate visual transduction. Defects in the ciliary machinery often result in improper formation of the outer segment of the retina and presents as retinal degeneration in patients [16 - 20].

Phosphoinositides and Inositol Phosphatases

Phosphoinositides, also referred to as phosphatidylinositol lipids, are ubiquitous phospholipid signaling molecules present in all mammalian cells [21]. Phosphoinositides are composed of a hydrophobic fatty acid and glycerol backbone, enabling the insertion into lipid membranes, linked to a soluble six sided inositol head group that may be phosphorylated at the D3, D4 and D5 positions, giving rise to seven different signaling molecules [22]. These signaling molecules regulate vesicular trafficking, cell proliferation and differentiation, protein synthesis and cytoskeletal rearrangements by acting as precursors to second messengers or by recruiting and activating phosphoinositide-binding effector proteins [7]. The intracellular levels of phosphoinositides are tightly regulated, both spatially and temporally, by a complicated and well choreographed interplay between phosphoinositide kinases and phosphatases (Fig. **1**).

Phosphoinositide kinases (*i.e.* phosphoinositide 3-kinase; PI3K) generate phosphoinositide second messengers such as phosphatidylinositol(3,4,5)-trisphosphate (PtdIns(3,4,5)P_3) by phosphorylation of phosphatidylinositol(4,5)-bisphosphate (PtdIns(4,5)P_2). PtdIns(4,5)P_2 is the most abundant phosphoinositide that serves as substrate for various phospholipases C, which generate diacylglycerol (DAG) and the soluble inositol Ins(1,4,5)P_3 by cleavage of PtdIns(4,5)P_2 [23]. Highly conserved inositol polyphosphate phosphatases hydrolyze their specific phosphorylated phosphoinositide substrates and are classified according to the position they dephosphorylate on the inositol ring.

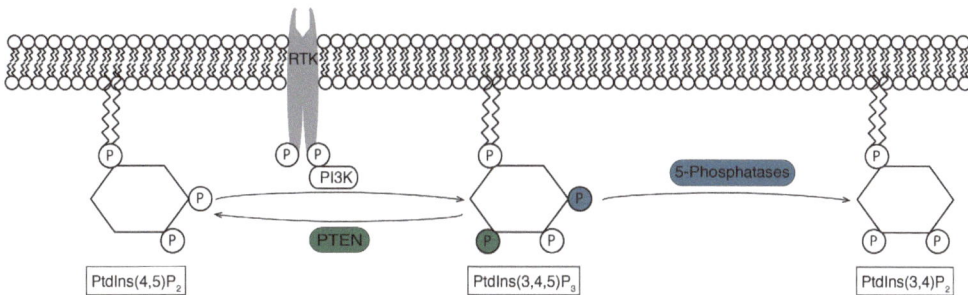

Fig. (1). Phosphoinositide kinases and phosphatases regulate intracellular levels of phosphoinositides. The binding of substrate to growth factor receptor tyrosine kinase (RTK) results in autophosphorylation on tyrosine residues of the receptor. Phosphoinositide 3-kinase (PI3K) activity is initiated by direct binding of PI3K to these phosphotyrosine residues, resulting in transient phosphorylation of PtdIns(4,5)P_2 to PtdIns(3,4,5)P_3. Inositol polyphosphate phosphatases such as the 3-phosphatase PTEN and 5-phosphatases (including OCRL, INPP5B and INPP5E) control phosphoinositide levels by removing a phosphate group from PtdIns(3,4,5)P_3. PTEN removes a phosphate group from the 3-position of the inositol ring generating PtdIns(4,5)P_2, whereas 5-phosphatases form PtdIns(3,4)P_2 by dephosphorylating the 5-position of the inositol ring.

The inositol polyphosphate 5-phosphatases (5-phosphatases) remove the phosphate group from the 5-position of the inositol ring in an Mg^{2+}-dependent mechanism [24]. Five known substrates for 5-phosphatases have been identified: the water soluble inositol phosphate substrates inositol 1,4,5-trisphosphate (Ins(1,4,5)P_3) and inositol 1,3,4,5-tetrakisphosphate (Ins(1,3,4,5)P_4), and the lipids PtdIns(3,5)P_2, PtdIns(3,4,5)P_3 and PtdIns(4,5)P_2. The 5-phosphatase family comprises ten mammalian members, which are classified into four groups based on substrate specificity [25]. Group I hydrolyzes only Ins(1,4,5)P_3 and Ins(1,3,4,5)P_4, group II hydrolyzes all known substrates, group III only hydrolyzes substrates with a phosphate group in the D3-position (*i.e.* PtdIns(3,4,5)P_3) and group IV is only active against PtdIns(3,4,5)P_3 and remains poorly understood. All members of the 5-phosphatases family share a conserved 300 amino acid catalytic 5-phosphatase domain. Additional protein-interaction domains confer unique specificity of 5-phosphatases depending on the cell types [26].

Dysfunctions of 5-phosphatases have been reported to be directly associated with a wide range of human diseases including cancer and diabetes [22, 24, 27]. Genetic mutations of several 5-phosphatases have been identified in ciliopathy syndromes or cilia-related syndromes [7, 28 - 30].

Importantly, many studies have revealed both inositol kinases and phosphatases play roles in cilia formation and ciliary function. For example, the inositol 1,3,4,5,6-pentakisphosphate 2-kinase (Ipk1) is essential in ciliary motility by generating inositol hexakisphosphate in zebrafish, whereas the inositol hexakisphosphate kinase-2 (IP6K2) acts as an effector of the Hhg pathway by producing inositol pyrophosphates (PP-IPs) (Fig. **2**) [31, 32]. This review will focus on the role of 5-phosphatases implicated in primary cilia and related human ocular diseases.

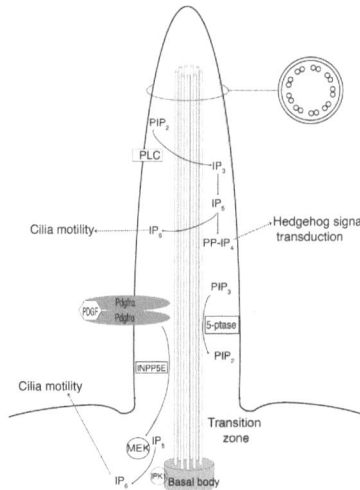

Fig. (2). Phosphoinositide signaling and cilia. Activation of phospholipase C (PLC) results in the initiation of soluble inositol polyphosphate (IP) messengers such as $Ins(1,4,5)P_3$ (IP_3) generated from $PtdIns(3,4)P_2$ (PIP_2). Sequentially, IP_3 is further phosphorylated producing more highly phosphorylated IPs such as inositol 1,3,4,5,6-pentakisphosphate (IP_5) and inositol hexakisphosphate (IP_6), which acts as an effector of ciliary motility. Other products that are generated are inositol pyrophosphates including PP-IP_4, which plays a role during sonic Hedgehog signaling. PIP_2 links the IP signaling pathway to the lipid phosphoinositide pathways and is the product of $PtdIns(3,4,5)P_3$ (PIP_3) dephosphorylation by 5-phosphatases including OCRL, INPP5B and INPP5E.

OCRL

The type II 5-phosphatase OCRL (also known as INPP5F or Oculocerebrorenal syndrome of Lowe) is a 105kDa protein that is highly expressed in kidney and brain, and also in anterior and posterior chambers of the eye [28, 33 - 35]. Its preferred substrate is $PtdIns(4,5)P_2$ and it also has catalytic activity towards $Ins(1,4,5)P_3$, $Ins(1,3,4,5)P_4$, $PtdIns(3,5)P_2$ and $PtdIns(3,4,5)P_3$. The OCRL protein is a multidomain protein with a central conserved 5-phosphatase catalytic domain, an ASH domain, a C-terminal RhoGAP-like domain and a N-terminal PH (pleckstrin homology) domain mediating phosphoinositide-binding activity [36]. Binding of phosphoinositides typically results in the recruitment of effector proteins to the membrane or the activation of effector proteins through activating conformational changes induced by phosphoinositides [37]. Specific phospho-inositide binding results in OCRL localization to various subcellular compart-ments including endosomes, lamellipodia, and Golgi apparatus, indicating OCRL's role in membrane trafficking, migration, cell adhesion, phagocytosis, and endocytosis [36 - 47].

The *OCRL* gene is mapped to the human chromosome Xq25 and contains 24 exons (23 of which are coding) [35]. There are more than 100 mutations reported in this gene [48, 49]. Most of them have been identified in Oculocerebrorenal syndrome of Lowe (Lowe syndrome), a very rare X-linked congenital disorder characterized by bilateral congenital glaucoma and cataracts, brain abnormalities and renal dysfunction [35, 50]. Congenital cataracts, the main ophthalmologic manifestation of Lowe syndrome, can be seen as early as 20-24 weeks of gestation and are almost always present at birth, and glaucoma is detected within the first year of patients' lives [51 - 53]. So far, about 22 mutations have been reported in patients with another rare X-linked chronic kidney disorder named Dent 2 disease, with the occurrence of Lowe syndrome symptoms, including mild intellectual impairment, hypotonia and cataract [54, 55]. Most disease-causing mutations are missense mutations in the 5-phosphatase domain; others are nonsense, deletion or insertion mutations in other regions and domains resulting in a premature truncation of OCRL protein, disruption of the protein's catalytic activity and, protein-protein interactions, a reduction in protein stability [56 - 58].

Recently, OCRL was shown to localize in basal body and axoneme of primary cilium, and to modulate ciliogenesis in renal epithelial cells and ocular-ciliated cell lines including retinal pigmented epithelial cells [28, 59, 60]. Moreover, cells isolated from Lowe syndrome patients presented shortened cilia length and decreased OCRL protein level [28, 60, 61]. Interestingly, missense mutations of OCRL in the phosphatase domain, such as F668V, D499A and D422A, block the interaction and recruitment of Rab8A to OCRL, resulting in defects of primary cilia length and ciliated cell numbers in ciliated RPE cells [28, 44, 62]. Mice with Ocrl knockout have no detectable phenotypes similar to Lowe syndrome or Dent 2 disease [63]; however, transgenic animals with INPP5B presented with renal phenotype in mice (see below). In a zebrafish model, *ocrl* knockdown embryos recapitulates typical ciliopathy features including defects of ocular development such as microphthalmia and microlentis [28, 60], both of which have been observed in patients with Lowe syndrome.

INPP5B

Structurally, the closest homologue of OCRL is the 75kDa type II inositol polyphosphate 5-phosphatase INPP5B, which hydrolyzes PtdIns(4,5)P$_2$, PtdIns(3,4,5)P$_3$, Ins(1,4,5)P$_3$ and Ins(1,3,4,5)P$_4$ [64]. The gene encoding INPP5B is located on human chromosome locus 1p34 and, interestingly, is flanked by numerous genes associated with genetic disorders involving lens development, kidney function and mental retardation, all of which are associated with Lowe Syndrome [26]. The INPP5B protein is comprised of a central 5-phosphatase catalytic domain, an ASH domain and a RHO GTPase-activating protein (GAP) like domain at the C-terminus. This domain organization has a 45% sequence identity with OCRL suggesting similar or overlapping functions [65, 66]. Indeed, INPP5B compensates the loss function of OCRL in some degrees. In mice, knockout of either Ocrl (*Ocrl$^{-/-}$*) or Inpp5b (*Inpp5b$^{-/-}$*) are phenotypically normal and fail to show the ocular manifestations of Lowe syndrome; double knockout of *Ocrl$^{-/-}$:Inpp5b$^{-/-}$* results in embryonic lethality [63, 67, 68]. The introduction of human INPP5B rescues the lethality of double knockout and leads to clinical renal and ocular features in Lowe syndrome and Dent 2 disease [33, 69, 70]. Similar to OCRL, INPP5B also has localizations in endosomes, phagosomes, lamellipodia, Golgi and primary cilia [33, 71 - 74]. INPP5B knockdown in zebrafish also resulted in cilia associated microphthalmia with dystrophic retina and thinner outer segments of retinal photoreceptors. Wildtype INPP5B partly rescues the cilia-related defects in ocrl zebrafish morphants [33]. Using human patient cells, many studies have demonstrated INPP5B rescues the defects caused by the loss function of OCRL in endocytic trafficking [75] and ciliogenesis [33], but not in cell migration [71] or clathrin-related membrane ruffles [76].

INPP5E

Another 5-phosphatase family member implicated in several human diseases is INPP5E (also known as inositol polyphosphate 5-phosphatase type IV), which was initially cloned by its 5-phosphatase type IV activity [77]. This 72kDa 5-phosphatase only hydrolyzes the membrane-associated lipid phosphates PtdIns(4,5)P$_2$, PtdIns(3,5)P$_2$ and PtdIns(3,4,5)P$_3$ [77, 78]. Structurally, INPP5E differs significantly from the other known 5-phosphatases with only 10-20% of amino acids being identical. It has an unusually high proline content in the N terminal region to facilitate its localization to the Golgi, whereas the C-terminal CAAX motif may mediate its ciliary localization (Fig. **3**) [29, 78]. In human tissues, INPP5E is expressed in several organs with the highest levels being detected in brain, heart, spleen pancreas and testis. Analysis of its subcellular localization revealed the presence of INPP5E on the cytoplasmic surface of the trans-Golgi and adjacent to the basal body and in the axoneme of primary cilia

[29, 78].

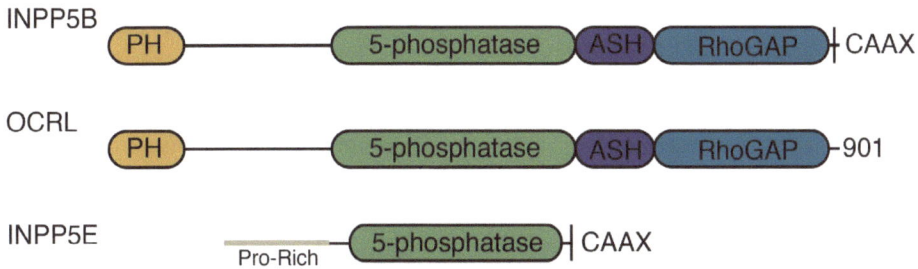

Fig. (3). Domain organization of the 5-phosphatases OCRL, INPP5B and INPP5E. The ASH domain is purple, the RhoGAP domain blue and the PH domain yellow.

The *INPP5E* gene is located on human chromosome 9q34.3. Mutations in *INPP5E* have been identified in a rare congenital disorder Joubert syndrome, characterized by midbrain malformation, retinitis pigmentosa, renal cysts, and polydactyly [29, 30, 79 - 88]. Thus far, most of the known Joubert syndrome mutations are missense mutations and cluster in the 5-phosphatase domain, suggesting that altering INPP5E enzymatic activities are required for cilia function. Three patient mutations (R621Q, Q627X, and C641R) fall within the C terminal domain of the protein with possible defects for lipid modification [89]. In addition to *INPP5E*, over twenty genes have been associated with Joubert syndrome and most of these gene products have been shown to localize to the base or axoneme of the primary cilia [84, 90 - 94]. A large mutation analysis for INPP5E of 483 probands revealed 12 different mutations in 17 probands from 11 Joubert syndrome families [89]. In MORM syndrome, a rare autosomal recessive disorder with similar features as another ciliopathy Bardet-Biedl syndrome [95], *INPP5E* nonsense mutations cause a deletion of the highly conserved C-terminal CAAX domain, which resulted in the failure of INPP5E to localize to primary cilium and reduced the stability of the primary cilium [29]. Phosphodiesterase 6D (PDE6D) is a prenyl-binding protein that has been shown to bind to INPP5E and a mutation in PDE6D has been found in a human Joubert patient with defect in targeting of farnesylated INPP5E to the cilia [96]. Recently, Humbert *et al.* showed that the ARL13B-INPP5E interaction plays an important role in ciliary targeting and mutations that affect this domain may result in Joubert syndrome [97]. Further ARL13B-INPP5E may form a functional network with PDE5D and centrosomal protein 164 (CEP164), with the former in the primary cilium and the latter two proteins in the centrosome and the distal appendage [97]. Separately Plotnikova *et al.* identified an interaction between INPP5E and Aurora Kinase A, which is an important regulator of mitosis and centrosomal assembly and stability [98]. Aurora Kinase A can phosphorylate INPP5E, which stimulates conversion of PtdIns(3,4,5)P$_3$ to PtdIns(3,4)P$_2$ and inhibition of AKT signaling cascade [98]. In *Inpp5e$^{-/-}$* mice, inhibition of Aurora Kinase A is able to restore normal ciliary stability, supporting the role of an upstream kinase in the regulation of inositol 5-phosphatase in primary cilia function.

In Joubert syndrome patients, ocular involvement commonly presents in the form of retinal dystrophy as a result of advancing degeneration of photoreceptor cells [99, 100]. This can present as a wide spectrum of clinical manifestations ranging from congenital retinal blindness to a variable degree of preservation of vision [99 - 101]. MORM syndrome patients present reduced visual acuity, cataracts and congenital retinal dystrophy in different decades of life [95]. An attempt to generate adult mice homozygous for the *Inpp5e* knockout failed because the animals died before or soon after birth. Analysis of the *Inpp5e$^{-/-}$* embryos revealed bilateral anophthalmos as well as polydactyly, polycystic kidneys and skeletal malformations. *Inpp5e* inactivation in adult mice results in complete absence of the retinal photoreceptor cell layer suggesting that the inactivation of *Inpp5e* leads to retinal dystrophy, which is one of the many features of ciliopathies [29]. In zebrafish, knockdown of *inpp5e* results in defects of ciliogenesis, microphthalmia and abnormal retinal development. Interestingly, all of these ciliary and cilia related phenotypes can be rescued by WT, not Joubert syndrome mutated, INPP5E [102]. During the preparation of this manuscript, two recent reports by Chavez *et al.* and Garcia-Gonzalo *et al.* show that PtdIns(4)P is the major ciliary phosphoinositide and INPP5E serves to dephosphorylate PtdIns(4,5)P$_2$ within the ciliary membrane [103, 104]. This may help to highlight the role of INPP5E as a regulator that defines the ciliary space. However, how the mutations in different inositol phosphatases result in disparate phenotypes remains to be examined.

CONCLUDING REMARKS

In the last two decades intensive research has contributed to a more detailed understanding of the function of inositol phosphatases, their role in regulating phosphoinositide levels and their importance in physiological processes in mammalian development and adult tissue homeostasis. Their importance in ciliogenesis has been established, but remains to be further investigated to understand how dysfunction of inositol phosphatases impacts ciliogenesis and contributes to the pathogenesis of numerous ciliopathies and other human diseases. Phosphatases of particular interest concerning retinal manifestations in ciliary disorders include the 5-phosphatases OCRL, INPP5B and INPP5E, all of which have been shown to play a role in ciliogenesis and embryonic ocular development. Further research will be required to determine the molecular pathways by which these phosphatases cause ocular manifestations in ciliopathies such as Lowe syndrome, Joubert syndrome and MORM syndrome.

CONFLICT OF INTEREST

The author (editor) declares no conflict of interest, financial or otherwise.

ACKNOWLEDGEMENTS

We like to thank Dr. Clark Wells for providing comments for this review.

REFERENCES

[1]   Cardenas-Rodriguez M, Badano JL. Ciliary biology: understanding the cellular and genetic basis of human ciliopathies. Am J Med Genet C Semin Med Genet 2009; 151C(4): 263-80.
[http://dx.doi.org/10.1002/ajmg.c.30227] [PMID: 19876935]

[2]   Fliegauf M, Benzing T, Omran H. When cilia go bad: cilia defects and ciliopathies. Nat Rev Mol Cell Biol 2007; 8(11): 880-93.
[http://dx.doi.org/10.1038/nrm2278] [PMID: 17955020]

[3]   Avasthi P, Marshall WF. Stages of ciliogenesis and regulation of ciliary length. Differentiation 2012; 83(2): S30-42.
[http://dx.doi.org/10.1016/j.diff.2011.11.015] [PMID: 22178116]

[4]   Baker K, Beales PL. Making sense of cilia in disease: the human ciliopathies. Am J Med Genet C Semin Med Genet 2009; 151C(4): 281-95.
[http://dx.doi.org/10.1002/ajmg.c.30231] [PMID: 19876933]

[5]   Ishikawa H, Marshall WF. Ciliogenesis: building the cell's antenna. Nat Rev Mol Cell Biol 2011; 12(4): 222-34.
[http://dx.doi.org/10.1038/nrm3085] [PMID: 21427764]

[6]   Yuan S, Sun Z. Expanding horizons: ciliary proteins reach beyond cilia. Annu Rev Genet 2013; 47: 353-76.
[http://dx.doi.org/10.1146/annurev-genet-111212-133243] [PMID: 24016188]

[7]   Conduit SE, Dyson JM, Mitchell CA. Inositol polyphosphate 5-phosphatases; new players in the regulation of cilia and ciliopathies. FEBS Lett 2012; 586(18): 2846-57.
[http://dx.doi.org/10.1016/j.febslet.2012.07.037] [PMID: 22828281]

[8]   Huangfu D, Liu A, Rakeman AS, Murcia NS, Niswander L, Anderson KV. Hedgehog signalling in the mouse requires intraflagellar transport proteins. Nature 2003; 426(6962): 83-7.
[http://dx.doi.org/10.1038/nature02061] [PMID: 14603322]

[9]   Simons M, Gloy J, Ganner A, *et al.* Inversin, the gene product mutated in nephronophthisis type II, functions as a molecular switch between Wnt signaling pathways. Nat Genet 2005; 37(5): 537-43.
[http://dx.doi.org/10.1038/ng1552] [PMID: 15852005]

[10] Schneider L, Clement CA, Teilmann SC, *et al.* PDGFRalphaalpha signaling is regulated through the primary cilium in fibroblasts. Curr Biol 2005; 15(20): 1861-6.
[http://dx.doi.org/10.1016/j.cub.2005.09.012] [PMID: 16243034]

[11] Ingham PW, Nakano Y, Seger C. Mechanisms and functions of Hedgehog signalling across the metazoa. Nat Rev Genet 2011; 12(6): 393-406.
[http://dx.doi.org/10.1038/nrg2984] [PMID: 21502959]

[12] Bai CB, Stephen D, Joyner AL. All mouse ventral spinal cord patterning by hedgehog is Gli dependent and involves an activator function of Gli3. Dev Cell 2004; 6(1): 103-15.
[http://dx.doi.org/10.1016/S1534-5807(03)00394-0] [PMID: 14723851]

[13] Corbit KC, Aanstad P, Singla V, Norman AR, Stainier DY, Reiter JF. Vertebrate Smoothened functions at the primary cilium. Nature 2005; 437(7061): 1018-21.

[http://dx.doi.org/10.1038/nature04117] [PMID: 16136078]

[14] Rohatgi R, Milenkovic L, Scott MP. Patched1 regulates hedgehog signaling at the primary cilium. Science 2007; 317(5836): 372-6.
[http://dx.doi.org/10.1126/science.1139740] [PMID: 17641202]

[15] Yildiz O, Khanna H. Ciliary signaling cascades in photoreceptors. Vision Res 2012; 75: 112-6.
[http://dx.doi.org/10.1016/j.visres.2012.08.007] [PMID: 22921640]

[16] Allen RA. Isolated cilia in inner retinal neurons and in retinal pigment epithelium. J Ultrastruct Res 1965; 12(5): 730-47.
[http://dx.doi.org/10.1016/S0022-5320(65)80058-2] [PMID: 5831058]

[17] Boycott BB, Hopkins JM. A neurofibrillar method stains solitary (primary) cilia in the mammalian retina: their distribution and age-related changes. J Cell Sci 1984; 66: 95-118.
[PMID: 6205006]

[18] Wheway G, Parry DA, Johnson CA. The role of primary cilia in the development and disease of the retina. Organogenesis 2014; 10(1): 69-85.
[http://dx.doi.org/10.4161/org.26710] [PMID: 24162842]

[19] Strauss O. The retinal pigment epithelium in visual function. Physiol Rev 2005; 85(3): 845-81.
[http://dx.doi.org/10.1152/physrev.00021.2004] [PMID: 15987797]

[20] Ramamurthy V, Cayouette M. Development and disease of the photoreceptor cilium. Clin Genet 2009; 76(2): 137-45.
[http://dx.doi.org/10.1111/j.1399-0004.2009.01240.x] [PMID: 19790290]

[21] Mitchell CA, Gurung R, Kong AM, Dyson JM, Tan A, Ooms LM. Inositol polyphosphate 5-phosphatases: lipid phosphatases with flair. IUBMB Life 2002; 53(1): 25-36.
[http://dx.doi.org/10.1080/15216540210815] [PMID: 12018404]

[22] Ooms LM, Horan KA, Rahman P, et al. The role of the inositol polyphosphate 5-phosphatases in cellular function and human disease. Biochem J 2009; 419(1): 29-49.
[http://dx.doi.org/10.1042/BJ20081673] [PMID: 19272022]

[23] Payrastre B, Missy K, Giuriato S, Bodin S, Plantavid M, Gratacap M. Phosphoinositides: key players in cell signalling, in time and space. Cell Signal 2001; 13(6): 377-87.
[http://dx.doi.org/10.1016/S0898-6568(01)00158-9] [PMID: 11384836]

[24] Hakim S, Bertucci MC, Conduit SE, Vuong DL, Mitchell CA. Inositol polyphosphate phosphatases in human disease. Curr Top Microbiol Immunol 2012; 362: 247-314.
[http://dx.doi.org/10.1007/978-94-007-5025-8_12] [PMID: 23086422]

[25] Majerus PW, Kisseleva MV, Norris FA. The role of phosphatases in inositol signaling reactions. J Biol Chem 1999; 274(16): 10669-72.
[http://dx.doi.org/10.1074/jbc.274.16.10669] [PMID: 10196133]

[26] Dyson JM, Fedele CG, Davies EM, Becanovic J, Mitchell CA. Phosphoinositide phosphatases: just as important as the kinases. Subcell Biochem 2012; 58: 215-79.
[http://dx.doi.org/10.1007/978-94-007-3012-0_7] [PMID: 22403078]

[27] McCrea HJ, De Camilli P. Mutations in phosphoinositide metabolizing enzymes and human disease. Physiology (Bethesda) 2009; 24: 8-16.
[http://dx.doi.org/10.1152/physiol.00035.2008] [PMID: 19196647]

[28] Luo N, West CC, Murga-Zamalloa CA, et al. OCRL localizes to the primary cilium: a new role for cilia in Lowe syndrome. Hum Mol Genet 2012; 21(15): 3333-44.
[http://dx.doi.org/10.1093/hmg/dds163] [PMID: 22543976]

[29] Jacoby M, Cox JJ, Gayral S, et al. INPP5E mutations cause primary cilium signaling defects, ciliary instability and ciliopathies in human and mouse. Nat Genet 2009; 41(9): 1027-31.
[http://dx.doi.org/10.1038/ng.427] [PMID: 19668215]

[30] Bielas SL, Silhavy JL, Brancati F, *et al.* Mutations in INPP5E, encoding inositol polyphosphate--phosphatase E, link phosphatidyl inositol signaling to the ciliopathies. Nat Genet 2009; 41(9): 1032-6.
[http://dx.doi.org/10.1038/ng.423] [PMID: 19668216]

[31] Sarmah B, Winfrey VP, Olson GE, Appel B, Wente SR. A role for the inositol kinase Ipk1 in ciliary beating and length maintenance. Proc Natl Acad Sci USA 2007; 104(50): 19843-8.
[http://dx.doi.org/10.1073/pnas.0706934104] [PMID: 18056639]

[32] Sarmah B, Wente SR. Inositol hexakisphosphate kinase-2 acts as an effector of the vertebrate Hedgehog pathway. Proc Natl Acad Sci USA 2010; 107(46): 19921-6.
[http://dx.doi.org/10.1073/pnas.1007256107] [PMID: 20980661]

[33] Luo N, Kumar A, Conwell M, Weinreb RN, Anderson R, Sun Y. Compensatory Role of Inositol 5-Phosphatase INPP5B to OCRL in Primary Cilia Formation in Oculocerebrorenal Syndrome of Lowe. PLoS One 2013; 8(6): e66727.
[http://dx.doi.org/10.1371/journal.pone.0066727] [PMID: 23805271]

[34] Olivos-Glander IM, Jänne PA, Nussbaum RL. The oculocerebrorenal syndrome gene product is a 105-kD protein localized to the Golgi complex. Am J Hum Genet 1995; 57(4): 817-23.
[PMID: 7573041]

[35] Attree O, Olivos IM, Okabe I, *et al.* The Lowe's oculocerebrorenal syndrome gene encodes a protein highly homologous to inositol polyphosphate-5-phosphatase. Nature 1992; 358(6383): 239-42.
[http://dx.doi.org/10.1038/358239a0] [PMID: 1321346]

[36] Mehta ZB, Pietka G, Lowe M. The cellular and physiological functions of the Lowe syndrome protein OCRL1. Traffic 2014; 15(5): 471-87.
[http://dx.doi.org/10.1111/tra.12160] [PMID: 24499450]

[37] Lemmon MA. Membrane recognition by phospholipid-binding domains. Nat Rev Mol Cell Biol 2008; 9(2): 99-111.
[http://dx.doi.org/10.1038/nrm2328] [PMID: 18216767]

[38] Faucherre A, Desbois P, Satre V, Lunardi J, Dorseuil O, Gacon G. Lowe syndrome protein OCRL1 interacts with Rac GTPase in the trans-Golgi network. Hum Mol Genet 2003; 12(19): 2449-56.
[http://dx.doi.org/10.1093/hmg/ddg250] [PMID: 12915445]

[39] Choudhury R, Diao A, Zhang F, *et al.* Lowe syndrome protein OCRL1 interacts with clathrin and regulates protein trafficking between endosomes and the trans-Golgi network. Mol Biol Cell 2005; 16(8): 3467-79.
[http://dx.doi.org/10.1091/mbc.E05-02-0120] [PMID: 15917292]

[40] Hyvola N, Diao A, McKenzie E, Skippen A, Cockcroft S, Lowe M. Membrane targeting and activation of the Lowe syndrome protein OCRL1 by rab GTPases. EMBO J 2006; 25(16): 3750-61.
[http://dx.doi.org/10.1038/sj.emboj.7601274] [PMID: 16902405]

[41] Erdmann KS, Mao Y, McCrea HJ, *et al.* A role of the Lowe syndrome protein OCRL in early steps of the endocytic pathway. Dev Cell 2007; 13(3): 377-90.
[http://dx.doi.org/10.1016/j.devcel.2007.08.004] [PMID: 17765681]

[42] McCrea HJ, Paradise S, Tomasini L, *et al.* All known patient mutations in the ASH-RhoGAP domains of OCRL affect targeting and APPL1 binding. Biochem Biophys Res Commun 2008; 369(2): 493-9.
[http://dx.doi.org/10.1016/j.bbrc.2008.02.067] [PMID: 18307981]

[43] Choudhury R, Noakes CJ, McKenzie E, Kox C, Lowe M. Differential clathrin binding and subcellular localization of OCRL1 splice isoforms. J Biol Chem 2009; 284(15): 9965-73.
[http://dx.doi.org/10.1074/jbc.M807442200] [PMID: 19211563]

[44] Swan LE, Tomasini L, Pirruccello M, Lunardi J, De Camilli P. Two closely related endocytic proteins that share a common OCRL-binding motif with APPL1. Proc Natl Acad Sci USA 2010; 107(8): 3511-6.
[http://dx.doi.org/10.1073/pnas.0914658107] [PMID: 20133602]

[45] Pirruccello M, Swan LE, Folta-Stogniew E, De Camilli P. Recognition of the F&H motif by the Lowe syndrome protein OCRL. Nat Struct Mol Biol 2011; 18(7): 789-95.
[http://dx.doi.org/10.1038/nsmb.2071] [PMID: 21666675]

[46] Addis M, Meloni C, Tosetto E, *et al.* An atypical Dent's disease phenotype caused by co-inheritance of mutations at CLCN5 and OCRL genes. Eur J Hum Genet 2013; 21(6): 687-90.
[http://dx.doi.org/10.1038/ejhg.2012.225] [PMID: 23047739]

[47] Trésaugues L, Silvander C, Flodin S, *et al.* Structural basis for phosphoinositide substrate recognition, catalysis, and membrane interactions in human inositol polyphosphate 5-phosphatases. Structure 2014; 22(5): 744-55.
[http://dx.doi.org/10.1016/j.str.2014.01.013] [PMID: 24704254]

[48] Hichri H, Rendu J, Monnier N, *et al.* From Lowe syndrome to Dent disease: correlations between mutations of the OCRL1 gene and clinical and biochemical phenotypes. Hum Mutat 2011; 32(4): 379-88.
[http://dx.doi.org/10.1002/humu.21391] [PMID: 21031565]

[49] Recker F, Zaniew M, Böckenhauer D, *et al.* Characterization of 28 novel patients expands the mutational and phenotypic spectrum of Lowe syndrome. Pediatr Nephrol 2015; 30(6): 931-43.
[http://dx.doi.org/10.1007/s00467-014-3013-2] [PMID: 25480730]

[50] Lowe CU, Terrey M, MacLACHLAN EA. Organic-aciduria, decreased renal ammonia production, hydrophthalmos, and mental retardation; a clinical entity. AMA Am J Dis Child 1952; 83(2): 164-84.
[PMID: 14884753]

[51] Loi M. Lowe syndrome. Orphanet J Rare Dis 2006; 1: 16.
[http://dx.doi.org/10.1186/1750-1172-1-16] [PMID: 16722554]

[52] Lewis RA, Nussbaum RL, Brewer ED. Lowe Syndrome. In: Pagon RA, Adam MP, Ardinger HH, Wallace SE, Amemiya A, Bean LJ, Eds. GeneReviews(R) Seattle WA. Seattle: University of Washington 1993.

[53] Walton DS, Katsavounidou G, Lowe CU. Glaucoma with the oculocerebrorenal syndrome of Lowe. J Glaucoma 2005; 14(3): 181-5.
[http://dx.doi.org/10.1097/01.ijg.0000158850.07732.05] [PMID: 15870597]

[54] Hoopes RR Jr, Shrimpton AE, Knohl SJ, *et al.* Dent Disease with mutations in OCRL1. Am J Hum Genet 2005; 76(2): 260-7.
[http://dx.doi.org/10.1086/427887] [PMID: 15627218]

[55] Shrimpton AE, Hoopes RR Jr, Knohl SJ, *et al.* OCRL1 mutations in Dent 2 patients suggest a mechanism for phenotypic variability. Nephron, Physiol 2009; 112(2): 27-36.
[http://dx.doi.org/10.1159/000213506] [PMID: 19390221]

[56] Hou X, Hagemann N, Schoebel S, *et al.* A structural basis for Lowe syndrome caused by mutations in the Rab-binding domain of OCRL1. EMBO J 2011; 30(8): 1659-70.
[http://dx.doi.org/10.1038/emboj.2011.60] [PMID: 21378754]

[57] Lin T, Orrison BM, Suchy SF, Lewis RA, Nussbaum RL. Mutations are not uniformly distributed throughout the OCRL1 gene in Lowe syndrome patients. Mol Genet Metab 1998; 64(1): 58-61.
[http://dx.doi.org/10.1006/mgme.1998.2687] [PMID: 9682219]

[58] Leahey AM, Charnas LR, Nussbaum RL. Nonsense mutations in the OCRL-1 gene in patients with the oculocerebrorenal syndrome of Lowe. Hum Mol Genet 1993; 2(4): 461-3.
[http://dx.doi.org/10.1093/hmg/2.4.461] [PMID: 8504307]

[59] Rbaibi Y, Cui S, Mo D, *et al.* OCRL1 modulates cilia length in renal epithelial cells. Traffic 2012; 13(9): 1295-305.
[http://dx.doi.org/10.1111/j.1600-0854.2012.01387.x] [PMID: 22680056]

[60] Coon BG, Hernandez V, Madhivanan K, *et al.* The Lowe syndrome protein OCRL1 is involved in

primary cilia assembly. Hum Mol Genet 2012; 21(8): 1835-47.
[http://dx.doi.org/10.1093/hmg/ddr615] [PMID: 22228094]

[61]   Luo N, Conwell MD, Chen X, *et al.* Primary cilia signaling mediates intraocular pressure sensation. Proc Natl Acad Sci USA 2014; 111(35): 12871-6.
[http://dx.doi.org/10.1073/pnas.1323292111] [PMID: 25143588]

[62]   Hagemann N, Hou X, Goody RS, Itzen A, Erdmann KS. Crystal structure of the Rab binding domain of OCRL1 in complex with Rab8 and functional implications of the OCRL1/Rab8 module for Lowe syndrome. Small GTPases 2012; 3(2): 107-10.
[http://dx.doi.org/10.4161/sgtp.19380] [PMID: 22790198]

[63]   Jänne PA, Suchy SF, Bernard D, *et al.* Functional overlap between murine Inpp5b and Ocrl1 may explain why deficiency of the murine ortholog for OCRL1 does not cause Lowe syndrome in mice. J Clin Invest 1998; 101(10): 2042-53.
[http://dx.doi.org/10.1172/JCI2414] [PMID: 9593760]

[64]   Jefferson AB, Majerus PW. Properties of type II inositol polyphosphate 5-phosphatase. J Biol Chem 1995; 270(16): 9370-7.
[http://dx.doi.org/10.1074/jbc.270.16.9370] [PMID: 7721860]

[65]   Matzaris M, O'Malley CJ, Badger A, Speed CJ, Bird PI, Mitchell CA. Distinct membrane and cytosolic forms of inositol polyphosphate 5-phosphatase II. Efficient membrane localization requires two discrete domains. J Biol Chem 1998; 273(14): 8256-67.
[http://dx.doi.org/10.1074/jbc.273.14.8256] [PMID: 9525932]

[66]   Speed CJ, Matzaris M, Bird PI, Mitchell CA. Tissue distribution and intracellular localisation of the 75-kDa inositol polyphosphate 5-phosphatase. Eur J Biochem 1995; 234(1): 216-24.
[http://dx.doi.org/10.1111/j.1432-1033.1995.216_c.x] [PMID: 8529643]

[67]   Hellsten E, Evans JP, Bernard DJ, Jänne PA, Nussbaum RL. Disrupted sperm function and fertilin beta processing in mice deficient in the inositol polyphosphate 5-phosphatase Inpp5b. Dev Biol 2001; 240(2): 641-53.
[http://dx.doi.org/10.1006/dbio.2001.0476] [PMID: 11784089]

[68]   Bernard DJ, Nussbaum RL. X-inactivation analysis of embryonic lethality in Ocrl wt/-; Inpp5b-/- mice. Mamm Genome 2010; 21(3-4): 186-94.
[http://dx.doi.org/10.1007/s00335-010-9255-9] [PMID: 20195868]

[69]   Bothwell SP, Farber LW, Hoagland A, Nussbaum RL. Species-specific difference in expression and splice-site choice in Inpp5b, an inositol polyphosphate 5-phosphatase paralogous to the enzyme deficient in Lowe Syndrome. Mamm Genome 2010; 21(9-10): 458-66.
[http://dx.doi.org/10.1007/s00335-010-9281-7] [PMID: 20872266]

[70]   Bothwell SP, Chan E, Bernardini IM, Kuo YM, Gahl WA, Nussbaum RL. Mouse model for Lowe syndrome/Dent Disease 2 renal tubulopathy. J Am Soc Nephrol 2011; 22(3): 443-8.
[http://dx.doi.org/10.1681/ASN.2010050565] [PMID: 21183592]

[71]   Coon BG, Mukherjee D, Hanna CB, Riese DJ II, Lowe M, Aguilar RC. Lowe syndrome patient fibroblasts display Ocrl1-specific cell migration defects that cannot be rescued by the homologous Inpp5b phosphatase. Hum Mol Genet 2009; 18(23): 4478-91.
[http://dx.doi.org/10.1093/hmg/ddp407] [PMID: 19700499]

[72]   Williams C, Choudhury R, McKenzie E, Lowe M. Targeting of the type II inositol polyphosphate 5-phosphatase INPP5B to the early secretory pathway. J Cell Sci 2007; 120(Pt 22): 3941-51.
[http://dx.doi.org/10.1242/jcs.014423] [PMID: 17956944]

[73]   Bohdanowicz M, Balkin DM, De Camilli P, Grinstein S. Recruitment of OCRL and Inpp5B to phagosomes by Rab5 and APPL1 depletes phosphoinositides and attenuates Akt signaling. Mol Biol Cell 2012; 23(1): 176-87.
[http://dx.doi.org/10.1091/mbc.E11-06-0489] [PMID: 22072788]

[74] Shin HW, Hayashi M, Christoforidis S, *et al.* An enzymatic cascade of Rab5 effectors regulates phosphoinositide turnover in the endocytic pathway. J Cell Biol 2005; 170(4): 607-18.
[http://dx.doi.org/10.1083/jcb.200505128] [PMID: 16103228]

[75] Noakes CJ, Lee G, Lowe M. The PH domain proteins IPIP27A and B link OCRL1 to receptor recycling in the endocytic pathway. Mol Biol Cell 2011; 22(5): 606-23.
[http://dx.doi.org/10.1091/mbc.E10-08-0730] [PMID: 21233288]

[76] Mao Y, Balkin DM, Zoncu R, *et al.* A PH domain within OCRL bridges clathrin-mediated membrane trafficking to phosphoinositide metabolism. EMBO J 2009; 28(13): 1831-42.
[http://dx.doi.org/10.1038/emboj.2009.155] [PMID: 19536138]

[77] Kisseleva MV, Wilson MP, Majerus PW. The isolation and characterization of a cDNA encoding phospholipid-specific inositol polyphosphate 5-phosphatase. J Biol Chem 2000; 275(26): 20110-6.
[http://dx.doi.org/10.1074/jbc.M910119199] [PMID: 10764818]

[78] Kong AM, Speed CJ, O'Malley CJ, *et al.* Cloning and characterization of a 72-kDa inositol-polyphosphate 5-phosphatase localized to the Golgi network. J Biol Chem 2000; 275(31): 24052-64.
[http://dx.doi.org/10.1074/jbc.M000874200] [PMID: 10806194]

[79] Joubert M, Eisenring JJ, Robb JP, Andermann F. Familial agenesis of the cerebellar vermis. A syndrome of episodic hyperpnea, abnormal eye movements, ataxia, and retardation. Neurology 1969; 19(9): 813-25.
[http://dx.doi.org/10.1212/WNL.19.9.813] [PMID: 5816874]

[80] Kumandas S, Akcakus M, Coskun A, Gumus H. Joubert syndrome: review and report of seven new cases. Eur J Neurol 2004; 11(8): 505-10.
[http://dx.doi.org/10.1111/j.1468-1331.2004.00819.x] [PMID: 15272893]

[81] Maria BL, Hoang KB, Tusa RJ, *et al.* "Joubert syndrome" revisited: key ocular motor signs with magnetic resonance imaging correlation. J Child Neurol 1997; 12(7): 423-30.
[http://dx.doi.org/10.1177/088307389701200703] [PMID: 9373798]

[82] Lee JE, Gleeson JG. Cilia in the nervous system: linking cilia function and neurodevelopmental disorders. Curr Opin Neurol 2011; 24(2): 98-105.
[http://dx.doi.org/10.1097/WCO.0b013e3283444d05] [PMID: 21386674]

[83] Brancati F, Dallapiccola B, Valente EM. Joubert Syndrome and related disorders. Orphanet J Rare Dis 2010; 5: 20.
[http://dx.doi.org/10.1186/1750-1172-5-20] [PMID: 20615230]

[84] Doherty D. Joubert syndrome: insights into brain development, cilium biology, and complex disease. Semin Pediatr Neurol 2009; 16(3): 143-54.
[http://dx.doi.org/10.1016/j.spen.2009.06.002] [PMID: 19778711]

[85] Saraiva JM, Baraitser M. Joubert syndrome: a review. Am J Med Genet 1992; 43(4): 726-31.
[http://dx.doi.org/10.1002/ajmg.1320430415] [PMID: 1341417]

[86] Parisi MA, Doherty D, Chance PF, Glass IA. Joubert syndrome (and related disorders) (OMIM 213300). Eur J Hum Genet 2007; 15(5): 511-21.
[http://dx.doi.org/10.1038/sj.ejhg.5201648] [PMID: 17377524]

[87] Parisi MA. Clinical and molecular features of Joubert syndrome and related disorders. Am J Med Genet C Semin Med Genet 2009; 151C(4): 326-40.
[http://dx.doi.org/10.1002/ajmg.c.30229] [PMID: 19876931]

[88] Gleeson JG, Keeler LC, Parisi MA, *et al.* Molar tooth sign of the midbrain-hindbrain junction: occurrence in multiple distinct syndromes. Am J Med Genet A 2004; 125A(2): 125-34.
[http://dx.doi.org/10.1002/ajmg.a.20437] [PMID: 14981712]

[89] Travaglini L, Brancati F, Silhavy J, *et al.* Phenotypic spectrum and prevalence of INPP5E mutations in Joubert syndrome and related disorders. Eur J Hum Genet 2013; 21(10): 1074-8.

[http://dx.doi.org/10.1038/ejhg.2012.305] [PMID: 23386033]

[90] Valente EM, Logan CV, Mougou-Zerelli S, *et al.* Mutations in TMEM216 perturb ciliogenesis and cause Joubert, Meckel and related syndromes. Nat Genet 2010; 42(7): 619-25.
[http://dx.doi.org/10.1038/ng.594] [PMID: 20512146]

[91] Gorden NT, Arts HH, Parisi MA, *et al.* CC2D2A is mutated in Joubert syndrome and interacts with the ciliopathy-associated basal body protein CEP290. Am J Hum Genet 2008; 83(5): 559-71.
[http://dx.doi.org/10.1016/j.ajhg.2008.10.002] [PMID: 18950740]

[92] Coene KL, Roepman R, Doherty D, *et al.* OFD1 is mutated in X-linked Joubert syndrome and interacts with LCA5-encoded lebercilin. Am J Hum Genet 2009; 85(4): 465-81.
[http://dx.doi.org/10.1016/j.ajhg.2009.09.002] [PMID: 19800048]

[93] Field M, Scheffer IE, Gill D, *et al.* Expanding the molecular basis and phenotypic spectrum of X-linked Joubert syndrome associated with OFD1 mutations. Eur J Hum Genet 2012; 20(7): 806-9.
[http://dx.doi.org/10.1038/ejhg.2012.9] [PMID: 22353940]

[94] Thauvin-Robinet C, Thomas S, Sinico M, *et al.* OFD1 mutations in males: phenotypic spectrum and ciliary basal body docking impairment. Clin Genet 2013; 84(1): 86-90.
[http://dx.doi.org/10.1111/cge.12013] [PMID: 23036093]

[95] Hampshire DJ, Ayub M, Springell K, *et al.* MORM syndrome (mental retardation, truncal obesity, retinal dystrophy and micropenis), a new autosomal recessive disorder, links to 9q34. Eur J Hum Genet 2006; 14(5): 543-8.
[http://dx.doi.org/10.1038/sj.ejhg.5201577] [PMID: 16493448]

[96] Thomas S, Wright KJ, Le Corre S, *et al.* A homozygous PDE6D mutation in Joubert syndrome impairs targeting of farnesylated INPP5E protein to the primary cilium. Hum Mutat 2014; 35(1): 137-46.
[http://dx.doi.org/10.1002/humu.22470] [PMID: 24166846]

[97] Humbert MC, Weihbrecht K, Searby CC, *et al.* ARL13B, PDE6D, and CEP164 form a functional network for INPP5E ciliary targeting. Proc Natl Acad Sci USA 2012; 109(48): 19691-6.
[http://dx.doi.org/10.1073/pnas.1210916109] [PMID: 23150559]

[98] Plotnikova OV, Seo S, Cottle DL, *et al.* INPP5E interacts with AURKA, linking phosphoinositide signaling to primary cilium stability. J Cell Sci 2015; 128(2): 364-72.
[http://dx.doi.org/10.1242/jcs.161323] [PMID: 25395580]

[99] Khan AO, Oystreck DT, Seidahmed MZ, *et al.* Ophthalmic features of Joubert syndrome. Ophthalmology 2008; 115(12): 2286-9.
[http://dx.doi.org/10.1016/j.ophtha.2008.08.005] [PMID: 19041481]

[100] Sturm V, Leiba H, Menke MN, *et al.* Ophthalmological findings in Joubert syndrome. Eye (Lond) 2010; 24(2): 222-5.
[http://dx.doi.org/10.1038/eye.2009.116] [PMID: 19461662]

[101] Valente EM, Brancati F, Dallapiccola B. Genotypes and phenotypes of Joubert syndrome and related disorders. Eur J Med Genet 2008; 51(1): 1-23.
[http://dx.doi.org/10.1016/j.ejmg.2007.11.003] [PMID: 18164675]

[102] Luo N, Lu J, Sun Y. Evidence of a role of inositol polyphosphate 5-phosphatase INPP5E in cilia formation in zebrafish. Vision Res 2012; 75: 98-107.
[http://dx.doi.org/10.1016/j.visres.2012.09.011] [PMID: 23022135]

[103] Garcia-Gonzalo FR, Phua SC, Roberson EC, *et al.* Phosphoinositides Regulate Ciliary Protein Trafficking to Modulate Hedgehog Signaling. Dev Cell 2015; 34(4): 400-9.
[http://dx.doi.org/10.1016/j.devcel.2015.08.001] [PMID: 26305592]

[104] Chávez M, Ena S, Van Sande J, de Kerchove d'Exaerde A, Schurmans S, Schiffmann SN. Modulation of ciliary phosphoinositide content regulates trafficking and sonic hedgehog signaling output. Dev Cell 2015; 34(3): 338-50.
[http://dx.doi.org/10.1016/j.devcel.2015.06.016] [PMID: 26190144]

CHAPTER 4

Understanding the Pathogenesis of Neurodegeneration in Diabetic Retinopathy (DR)

Shahna Shahulhameed[1], Subhabrata Chakrabarti[1], Jay K. Chhablani[2] and **Inderjeet Kaur[1,*]**

[1] *Brien Holden Eye Research Centre, LV Prasad Eye Institute Hyderabad, India*

[2] *Smt. Kannuri Santhamma Centre for Vitreo Retinal diseases, LV Prasad Eye Institute Hyderabad, India*

Abstract: Diabetic Retinopathy (DR) is the leading cause of irreversible global vision loss. It affects the entire neurovascular unit of the retina, along with gradual neuro-degeneration and neuroinflammation. DR has primarily been considered a microvasculature complication of diabetes, a well-known metabolic disorder. However, recent studies have reported the presence of neurodegenerative changes in the retina of DR patients prior to clinical manifestations. In this review, we have compiled clinical, histopathological, biochemical and genetic evidences that suggest a role of neurodegeneration in DR progression and pathogenesis. These studies indicated neural changes in the retina that have lead to microvascular alterations. Furthermore, the mechanisms underlying the neural changes can help identify drug targets for effective management of the disease, which in turn will help reduce the burden of visual impairments caused by DR.

Keywords: Degenerative disease, Diabetes, Inflammation, Neurons, Retina.

NEURODEGENERATION

Neurodegeneration can be defined as the degenerative changes (both structural and functional) in neurons that lead to progressive loss of neuronal function whilst promoting their death through apoptosis or other mechanisms like autophagy and necrosis [1]. Neuronal damages are irreversible and show detrimental effects on the human body. Neurodegenerative changes include an increased rate of cell death and proliferation of macroglial population (known as reactive gliosis and recognized by the increased expression of glial fibrillary acidic protein (GFAP) and microglial activation [2, 3]. Neurodegeneration has been implicated in the pathogenesis of central nervous system diseases like Parkinson's, Alzheimer's

* **Corresponding author Inderjeet Kaur:** Scientist, Brien Holden Eye Research Centre, KAR Campus, L.V. Prasad Eye Institute, Road No. 2, Banjara Hills, Hyderabad- 500034, India; Tel: +91-40-30612508; E-mails: inderjeet@lvpei.org; ikaurs@gmail.com

and Huntington's disease [4, 5]. The eye is also vulnerable to neurodegenerative changes, as found in the pathogenesis of vision threatening diseases such as glaucoma, retinitis pigmentosa and age related macular degeneration [6 - 8]. However, neuronal damage has not been documented in diabetic retinopathy (DR) [9].

DIABETIC RETINOPATHY

Diabetes is one of the major causes of socio-economic burdens in the developing world. It is comprised of a group of metabolic diseases that affect multiple organs. The retina can be severely affected by the diabetic changes, leading to catastrophic loss of vision (termed Diabetic Retinopathy). DR manifests as damaged vascular as well as neuronal networks causing vitreous hemorrhage, microaneurysms, lipid exudates, cotton wool spots, macular edema and abnormal neovascularization [10].

A recent population-based study (2012) estimated the overall global prevalence of DR to be 34.6%. This number is increasing exponentially [11]. The duration of diabetes and glucose levels are major risk factors that determine the prevalence of DR [12]. The Wisconsin Epidemiologic Study of DR observed that 80% of patients with diabetes developed retinopathy within 15 years of its onset. The study also noted that the prevalence of advanced stage of DR was 67% in people with a longer duration of diabetes (>35 years), while it occurred in only 1.2% of people with shorter disease duration (<10 years) [13]. According to a WHO report, the occurrence of diabetes in India reached 31.1 million people. The WHO report also claims that this number will double each year [14]. The 2007 Andhra Pradesh Eye Disease Study (APEDS) in Southern India suggested an estimate of around 2.77 million people with DR and nearly 0.07 million people with severe DR [15].

Complications of Diabetic Retinopathy

DR is classified in two categories: non-proliferative diabetic retinopathy (NPDR) and proliferative diabetic retinopathy (PDR). These categories are based on the detectable changes in the retinal microvasculature. NPDR represents the earliest stage of DR. In patients with poor diabetic control, NPDR slowly progresses to the severe proliferative PDR stage. In mild NPDR, patients show one microaneurysm or dot blot hemorrhage in fundus quadrants. In severe NPDR, hemorrhage, venous bleeding and abnormalities in intra-retinal microvasculature are commonly observed [16].

In PDR, the ischemic retina releases growth factors like the vascular endothelial growth factor (VEGF) that induce the proliferation of abnormal vessels in the retina [17]. The newly formed vessels known as neovessels are fragile and tend to bleed at any time, causing vitreous hemorrhage. These neovessels create tractions in the retina as well as the detachment of the retina from the choroid. Neovascular glaucoma is also a vision-threatening complication of PDR, which is caused by the formation of new vessels, which can block the normal aqueous humor flow in the anterior chamber of the eye [18]. Another major factor of vision loss in DR is diabetic macular edema (DME), which is characterized by the accumulation of leaked fluids from the retinal capillaries in the macula, area of central vision [19].

Therapeutic approaches for DR depend upon the severity of the complications in patients. The most widely used approach during early disease stage is retinal laser photocoagulation [20]. This treatment seals leaked vessels, which redirects the blood supply and reduces overall oxidative damage.

Lately, anti-VEGF therapy has become a preferred strategy in the management of DME. VEGF is essential for many physiological functions in the retina. It plays a major role in vasculogenesis and neurogenesis. It is also an important neuroprotective agent in the retina. However, a side effect of anti-VEGF therapy is neurodegeneration [21].

NEURODEGENERATION IN DIABETIC RETINOPATHY

The retina is a highly metabolically active tissue in the eye. It is a well-organized laminated structure of multiple cell types (Fig. **1**). The vertebrate retina contains two synaptic layers intercalated between three nuclear layers: outer nuclear layer (ONL), inner nuclear layer (INL) and ganglion cell layer (GCL). The ONL contains rod and cone photoreceptor nuclei, whereas the INL is composed of horizontal, bipolar and amacrine cell nuclei. The GCL contains the nuclei of retinal ganglion cells (RGC) and displaced amacrine cells [22]. The retinal nerve fiber layer (RNFL) forms the innermost layer and is composed of axons of the ganglion cells. The nourishment to neuronal cells in the retina is provided through the blood vessels which are organized in a specific pattern in the retina. The communication between the blood vessels and neuronal cells in the retina is maintained by two types of glial cells: microglia and macroglia [23]. This entire cellular network in the retina gets compromised in DR. A majority of the studies on DR is primarily focused on the changes in the microvasculature of the retina. However, the neuronal damage in DR pathogenesis has largely been overlooked. Various preclinical and clinical studies have also provided plenty of evidence for neuronal damage in diabetic eyes, which is discussed in the next section.

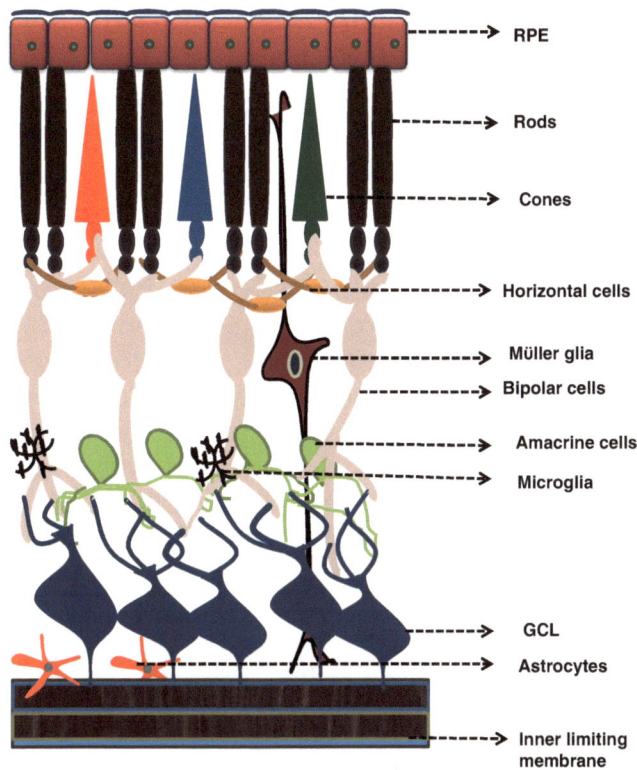

Fig. (1). Schematic representation of the retina: The vertebrate retina contains ten layers with 5 different types of neurons such as photoreceptors, horizontal cells, bipolar cells, amacrine cells and ganglion cell. The RPE provides nutrients to the photoreceptors. The glial cells are positioned critically between the cells of the vasculature and neurons, which maintain retinal homeostasis. The ganglion cells (GCs) receive the information from photoreceptors through bipolar and amacrine cells.

Clinical Evidences of Neurodegeneration in Diabetic Retinopathy

Several clinical studies have been conducted to understand the involvement of neuronal loss in DR pathogenesis. Evidences for RGC loss and reduced color and contrast sensitivity in diabetic eyes prior to the onset of retinopathy points towards neuronal damage in the retina [24 - 27]. Retinal imaging using spectral-domain optical coherence tomography (SD-OCT) has depicted the loss of RGCs in diabetic patients who have not yet developed any clinical symptoms of DR. Progressive loss of RGCs was also noted in moderate and severe DR [28]. A reduction in RNFL thickness was also reported in patients with diabetes and no DR [29]. A strong correlation between thinning of the ganglion cell-inner plexiform layer (GCIPL) and poor visual acuity was also seen in diabetic maculopathy patients. In these patients, the region in the retina responsible for central vision (called macula) is damaged due to the accumulation of fluid from the leaky vessels in the retina [30]. Likewise, the assessment of the GCIPL and RNFL in eyes of patients with different stages of DR identified a generalized thinning of the GCL and RNFL in all stages of DR as well as in the diabetic patients with no DR [31]. The thinning of GCL and RNFL seen in patients with minimal DR and vascular damage could be due to apoptosis of RGCs and further suggests that chronic neuronal damage precedes vascular damage in DR [32].

Animal Models of Neuronal Damage in Diabetic Retinopathy

Several studies employed animal models of DR to examine the early neuronal damage. Significant neural apoptosis within one month of the onset of diabetes and reduction of RGCs after long-term exposure to diabetes were noted in a rat model [33]. In Ins2^{Akita} mice, the thinning of the INL was observed due to the loss of bipolar, amacrine and horizontal cell bodies. Reduction in IPL thickness [34] and the loss of cholinergic and dopaminergic signaling in the retina were also associated with severe vision loss [35, 36]. The reduction of tyrosine hydroxylase immunoreactive amacrine cells, responsible for dopaminergic neurotransmission were seen in the immunohistochemical analysis in streptozotocin-induced male Sprague-Dawley rats [37].

The functional and pathological alterations of the neurosensory retina of the db/db (BKS/DB−/−) diabetic mice models were studied by pattern electroretinography (ERG), OCT, fundus fluorescein angiography (FFA) and immunohistochemistry using neuroinflammatory markers expressed by activated microglia. Significant alterations were seen in the ERG of diabetic compared to the non-diabetic mice. OCT revealed the thinning of the dorsal and temporal retina in the diabetic mice. These mice displayed significantly higher apoptosis of the RGCs along with the presence of neuroinflammatory markers. However, no vascular damages were observed on FFA, confirming that neural changes precede the vascular damage, and neuroinflammation is one of the earlier events in DR pathology [38].

Evidence from Pathophysiology of Affected Tissue

The immunohistopathology of retinal tissues from diabetic individuals revealed a higher glial reactivity, as suggested by the higher expression of GFAP compared to the control and noticeable growth of Müller glia into the occluded retinal vessels [39]. Müller cells are the major glia in the retina. They span the entire retina with long extensions. These cells play a major role in maintaining retinal homeostasis mainly by regulating the levels of neurotransmitters like glutamate. The effect of diabetes on Müller cells was studied by staining the major proteins in the Müller glia, such as glutamine synthetase (GS), GFAP and anti-apoptotic protein Bcl2 in human post-mortem retinal eyes of diabetics and of controls. This study could not find major changes in the expression of GS and Bcl2 in the Müller glia, however, significant upregulation of GFAP was observed throughout the Müller glia extensions [40]. Further, a significant drop in RGC count along with the presence of abnormal dendritic structures in the retina were noticed in rat models [41].

MECHANISMS OF NEURONAL DAMAGE IN DIABETIC RETINA

The structural and functional alterations of the neurons are the major manifestations of any neurodegenerative condition. A study by Barber *et al.,* used a rat model of DR and evaluated relative retinal layers thickness of diabetic rats *versus* the age-matched control. Significant reduction of the thickness of the INL and IPL was observed in the diabetic rats compared to controls. Additionally, a 10% reduction in the ganglion cell density in the retina was seen in diabetic rats. The diabetic retina displayed increased terminal deoxynucleotidyl transferase dUTP nick end labeling (TUNEL) positivity as compared to controls at all time periods. Further, minimal co-localization of TUNEL positive cells and Von Willebrand factor (vWF) stained endothelial cells indicated that endothelial cells were not apoptotic in the early stages of diabetes. Most of the TUNEL positive cells were seen in the GCL. Similar data were obtained with human tissue samples [33]. Martin *et al.,* also used a similar approach in diabetic mice and found 20-25% reduction in ganglion cell count after 14 weeks of diabetes. A higher number of TUNEL positive cells along with the active caspase-3, which plays a central role in apoptotic DNA fragmentation was seen in diabetic retina, further emphasized that neuronal death in DR is mediated by apoptosis [42].

The presence of apoptotic molecules in the diabetic retina provided the evidence for apoptosis to be one of the major mechanisms of neuronal damage under the hyperglycemic state. But the trigger for apoptosis has not been well established. Several studies attempted to identify the major apoptotic molecules in the diabetic retina by IHC using various known markers of apoptosis. Upon comparing the retinas of diabetic mice *versus* non-diabetic controls, a weak GFAP, Bcl2 and extracellular-signal-regulated *kinases 1/2*(ERK1/2) expression was noted in the controls, whereas a higher expression of these markers was seen in the RNFL and GCL along with the accumulation of apoptotic molecules like caspase-3, Fas, Fas L and Bax in the diabetic retinas. The strong expression of ERK1/2 in glial cell nuclei in diabetic retina indicated the protection of glial cells in diabetic induced damage. The presence of Fas in the glial cells suggested the glial induced apoptosis of ganglion cells [43].

In another study, the key molecules involved in the apoptosis and survival of the neuroretina were studied using human retinal diabetic and non-diabetic tissue samples. This study also identified FasL, a pro-apoptotic molecule in the neuroretina of the diabetic subjects. FasL is also known to induce the formation of death-inducing signaling complex (DISC) through the death receptor pathway and by recruiting caspase-8. Additionally, molecules such as Bim and Caspase-3 that are involved in the apoptosis *via* the mitochondrial pathways had higher expression in the diabetic neuroretina. This study clearly proved the involvement of death receptor pathway in neural apoptosis in DR [44].

Electron microscopy studies of diabetic rat retinas revealed the loss of photoreceptors in the ONL after 24 weeks of diabetes, but the degenerative changes such as myelinated and multi-vesicular mitochondrial features appeared within 1 week of diabetes [45]. Somatostatin, a neuromodulator as well as an antiangiogenic factor produced by neural cells of the retina, was downregulated in diabetic retinas [46]. This suggested that reduction of somatostatin could be an early event in DR that damaged the neural retina [47].

Piano *et al.*, demonstrated a role of autophagy in DR by examining the progression of retinal dysfunction in streptozotocin-induced diabetic C57BL/6J mice at an interval of 4, 8 and 12 weeks. There was a significant reduction in the amplitudes of scotopic "a" and "b" waves due to rod cell damage in diabetic mice compared to the controls. Synaptic degeneration was seen mainly after 8 and 12 weeks of diabetes and a significant reduction in deep plexus vessel complexity was observed [48].

Inflammation and Neuronal Damage

DR being a metabolic disorder has also been considered an inflammatory disorder. Support for this hypothesis comes from previous studies demonstrating significant correlation with the symptoms of inflammation such as hemorrhage, edema, leukocyte adhesion. Moreover, inflammation plays a major role in the progression of DR [49]. The analyses of vitreous samples in various studies identified proinflammatory and inflammatory cytokines such as *Tumor necrosis factor* alpha (TNFα), Interleukin-1 beta (IL-1β), Interleukin-6 (IL-6), Interleukin-8 (IL-8), Monocyte chemoattractant protein-1(MCP-1) *etc.* [50 - 52].

Another important component of inflammation is the complement pathway. Retinal microglial cells, RPE and the complement system comprise the retinal innate immune system. Excessive complement activation has been implicated in the pathogenesis of various ocular conditions, such as corneal neovascularization, age-related macular degeneration and other retinopathies [53]. Accumulation of complement components was seen in the choriocapillaris of diabetic patients. The inflammatory reactions in the retina further activate other glial cells in the retina and damage the neurosensory retina. Inflammation and associated gliosis are involved in the pathogenesis of neurodegenerative, diseases like Parkinson's and

Alzheimer's [54]. Thus, inflammation, glial cell activation and functional alteration of the retina neurons, especially thinning of the RNFL by ganglion cell loss point to a chronic neurodegeneration in DR.

Glial Activation, A Cellular Mechanism of Neuronal Damage

The macroglial and microglial populations in the retina are involved in retinal homeostasis. Several studies have shown that gliosis and increased expression of GFAP are indicators of neuronal damage [44, 55]. The inflammatory environment and the presence of markers of glial activation indicate a role of glial cells in neuroinflammation and vascular damage in DR. Under ischemic stress or altered microenvironment, both the macroglia and microglia play independent roles in maintaining retinal homeostasis and causing damage.

Astrocytes and Müller glia are the major macroglial population in the retina. Unlike other cells types, Müller glia span the retina with its long stem like extensions, *i.e.* they contact all retinal neuronal cell types. The Müller cells contain neurotransmitter receptors, and their interaction with neurons plays a crucial role in retinal development. Calcium plays a significant role in bidirectional signaling between the neuroglial cells. In response to various neurotransmitters, Müller cells show highest calcium transients (rise of calcium from intracellular spaces) in the developing retina. The calcium transients was reduced upon neuronal development due to changes in neurotransmitter release, indicating the role of neuroglial crosstalk during development and homeostasis of the retina [56]. Furthermore, there is an increase in intracellular calcium in mechanically stimulated astrocytes with the simultaneous release of glutamate [57].

Gene expression analysis of Müller glia in streptozotocin-induced rats revealed an increase in the expression of the major proteins associated with gliosis, such as GFAP and Ceruloplasmin [58]. Inflammation can also alter the function of Müller glia by changing its function of neuroprotection. High glucose stress to Müller glia caused glucose toxicity by inducing the production of IL-1β and IL-6. IL-1β further caused apoptosis of the Müller glia by caspase-1 dependent mechanism [59]. The Müller glial cells in the retina also play a major role in maintaining glutamate levels [60]. Glutamate is a major excitatory neurotransmitter and is released from the presynaptic neuronal terminal. The released glutamate is taken up by the glutamate transporter in the Müller glia, where it is converted to glutamine and transported to the retinal neurons. However, if not cleared from the extracellular space, glutamine acts as a neurotoxin [61]. Various animal model and patient studies have revealed elevated glutamate levels in diabetic eyes [62]. The elevated levels of glutamate have deleterious effects on the RGCs. Higher levels of glutamate were also found in vitreous of patients with DR [63].

Glial reactivity and elevation of glutamate levels have been shown to cause neural apoptosis. Lieth *et al.,* used streptozotocin-induced diabetic rats to study the glial reactivity in the early course of diabetes. A remarkable increase in GFAP was noted after 3 months of diabetes in rats compared to their age matched control by two-site ELISA, indicating the macroglial activation in diabetic retina [63].

The ability of the glial cells to metabolize glutamate is dependent on the receptors which are assigned for glutamate uptake. L-glutamate/L-aspartate transporter (GLAST) is a major glutamate transporter present in the macroglial population of the retina. Its major role is to remove the glutamate from the extracellular space and thus, to protect the neurons, especially RGCs [64]. The activity of GLAST in Müller glia under hyperglycemic condition was analyzed by electrophysiological methods. A significant decrease in GLAST activity was found in Müller glia isolated from diabetic rats, indicating hyperglycemia-induced oxidative stress affected the ability of glutamate uptake in Müller glia [61].

Glutamine synthetase, an important enzyme specifically present in Müller cells is involved in the conversion of glutamate to glutamine. In the streptozotocin-induced diabetic rat model, reduced activity of this enzyme was noted in the Müller glia [65]. Thus, the altered receptor function, gliosis, and reduction in the enzyme activity cause glutamate excitotoxicity and neuronal damage.

Microglia

Microglia represents the resident immune cells of the central nervous system (CNS), which are distributed throughout the inner retinal layers. The resting microglia maintains a ramified shape, but in the case of any homeostatic disturbance in the retina like diabetes or ischemia, these cells sense the signals and attain an amoeboid shape (activated microglia). Microglial activation is an invariable factor of neuronal damage and chronic neurodegeneration, indicating its detrimental role in DR [66]. Upon activation, these cells secreted various cytokines such as such as TNF-α and IL-1β [67]. Inflammatory conditions and hyperglycemia activate microglia and stimulate inflammation, and cause vascular breakdown leading to glial dysfunction and neuronal death [68].

The comparison of microglial morphology in patients with pre-proliferative and proliferative retinopathies compared with normal subjects using a specific cluster of differentiation (CD) markers such as CD68, CD45, and human leukocyte antigen-D related (HLA-DR) antigens revealed markedly increased and hypertrophic microglia during disease. In exudative retinopathy cases, increased cell number and labeling intensity of microglia were reported whereas, in pre-proliferative DR patients, the microglia became hypertrophic and clustered around the peripheral region of cotton wool spots and the dilated venules. Likewise, in proliferative retinopathy, the microglial clusters were observed around the new vessels in the nerve fiber layer of the retina. The new vessels were heavily surrounded by labeled microglial cells in the region of retinal vascularization breaking through the internal limiting membrane and further grown into the vitreous cavity [69].

Apart from microglial activation, microglial trafficking is another feature in diabetic eyes. Omri *et al.,* compared the distribution pattern of Iba1 positive cells in diabetic rat *versus* control. They reported numerous positive cells in the retina and the subretinal space. Interestingly, RPE breakdown was observed in diabetic rats with the formation of an intracellular pore [70]. Various factors and mechanisms can activate microglia during the early phase of DR. The accumulation of advanced glycation end (AGE) products affects multiple organs. A study by Ibrahim *et al.,* correlated the AGE product such as amygdala glycated protein and microglial activation in diabetic eyes. The deposition of AGE was associated with increased microglial activation and TNFα level in diabetic rat retinas. The activation of microglia by AGE was mediated by phosphorylation of Mitogen-activated protein kinases (MAPK) [71].

The cytokine released from the microglial cells further caused a neuronal damage. A study conducted by Cardona *et al.,* tried to understand the microglial activation and cytokine release and its association with the neuronal damage in DR. A significant reduction of Fractalkine in diabetic mice retina and subsequent increase of microglial activation was observed. Fractalkine is a neuronal membrane molecule and controls microglial activation by the CX3C chemokine receptor 1 (CX3CR1) present on microglia. Fractalkine also acts as an inhibitory signal on microglia, whereby its reduced expression leads to the production of neurotoxic cytokine IL-1β that further induces the RGC death [72].

Role of Oxidative Stress in Neuroinflammation and Degeneration

Ischemia due to hyperglycemia is one of the major factors involved in DR. Ischemia causes oxidative stress and leads to the generation of reactive oxygen species (ROS), which cause mitochondrial dysfunction by superoxide production [73, 74]. The ROS induces DNA damage, membrane permeability and autophagy [75]. The RGCs contain numerous mitochondria because of its higher energy requirement, hence are susceptible to the oxidative stress and autophagy [76]. The oxidative stress also causes activation of various inflammatory pathways like polyol pathway, PKC pathway, AGE pathways, Nuclear factor kappa-light-cha-n-enhancer of activated B cells (NF-κB) activation [77].

Another important feature of hypoxic stress is the production of VEGF. Müller cells are the major source of VEGF in the retina. Conditional ablation of VEGF in mice led to reduced inflammation, leukocytosis and decreased vascular leakage [78]. These observations indicated the dual role of Müller glia in vascular proliferation by providing VEGF and neuronal damage by secreting inflammatory molecules (Fig. **2**).

Anti-VEGF drugs can be used as a treatment strategy. However, VEGF being a neuroprotectant, its normal levels are required for neuronal survival [21, 79].

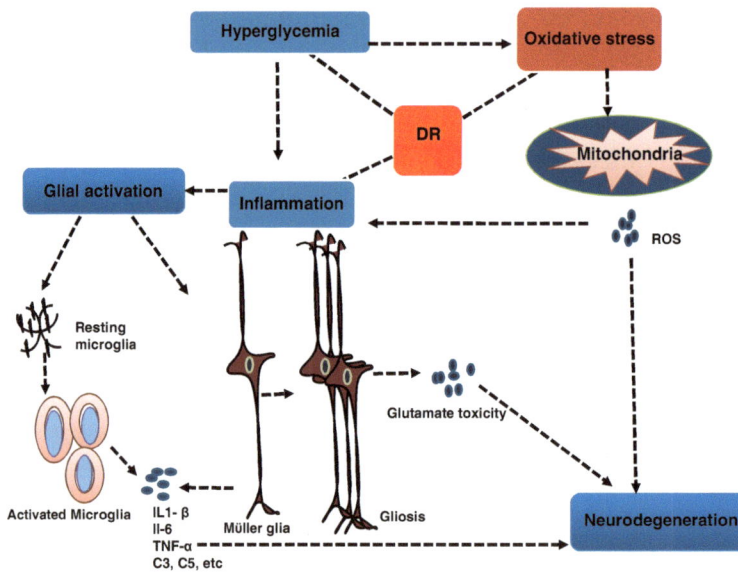

Fig. (2). Cellular Mechanism of neurodegeneration in Diabetic retinopathy: The altered microenvironment of diabetes induces multiple effects on the retina by various mechanisms. High glucose induces mitochondrial damage and ROS generation. These changes induce the activation of the glial population and lead to the secretion of various inflammatory molecules. Accumulation of glutamate due to Müller glia dysfunction, inflammatory cytokines and other various unfavorable factors in the retina affect the normal neuronal function and lead to degeneration of neurons.

Genetic Factors in Diabetic Retinopathy

Along with the altered cellular mechanisms, genetic predisposition also contributes to DR. However, only a few candidate genes have been associated with DR. The gene that codes for aldose reductase, Aldo-Keto Reductase Family 1, Member B1 (*AKR1B1*), a major regulator of the polyol pathway, is one of the important genes in diabetes-associated complications like nephropathy [80]. The polyol pathway plays a role in the apoptosis of retinal neurons in DR during high threshold hyperglycemic condition [81].

The Diabetes Control and Complications Trial (DCCT)/Epidemiology of Diabetes Interventions and Complications (EDIC) genetics study identified multiple variants in *VEGF* that were associated with severe diabetic retinopathy [82]. The genes involved in apoptosis and retinal permeability at 1 and 3 months of diabetes were studied using diabetic rats by microarray analysis. These studies revealed significant alteration in the expression of 32 genes in diabetic animals. These included Doublecortin-Like Kinase 1(*DCAMKL1*) and peptide transporter *PEPT2* [83]. *DCAMKL1* encoded protein Doublecortin is required for the regulation of microtubule polymerization and is highly expressed in the GCL [84]. *PEPT2* is involved in peptide transport across the membrane and is expressed in the Müller cells and astrocytes [85]. Another important finding was increased expression of proinflammatory genes, such as complement component 1 inhibitor (*C1-INH*), CC motif receptor 5 (*CCR5*), *CD44* and chitinase 3-like 1 (*CHI3L1*) [83].

Evidence from Proteomic Analysis of Vitreous Humor in Diabetic Retinopathy

Several vitreous proteomic studies were conducted to identify differentially expressed proteins under hyperglycemic condition. Interestingly, the majority of proteins that were dysregulated in the vitreous of PDR patients are responsible for neurodegeneration. Some of these proteins are summarized in Table **1**. Notable among these were Crystallins, Vimentin, GFAP, C3, C1, MCP-1, and PEDF [86 - 89]. Retinal expression of β and γ crystallins pertains to vascular remodeling during the development [90]. Upregulation of β and γ crystallins was also seen in neurons and cells involved in ganglion cell axon regrowth. Upregulation of α crystallin with an increase in the vimentin and GFAP in the early disease stages suggested a role of Müller glia cells in disease pathogenesis [86]. Complements are shown to be synthesized by RPE, Müller glia and microglia in the retina and in turn activate the microglia further leading to the upregulation of angiogenic proteins and downregulation of antiangiogenic proteins [91, 92].

Table 1. Proteins associated with the development of diabetic retinopathy.

Sl. No	Protein	Functions	Findings in DR	Inference	Ref.
1	Crystallin	Neuronal protectant	Increased expression of Crystallin isoform in DR, especially γ-Crystallin in RGC and β in other retinal neurons	To protect neurons from inflammation associated damage in DR	[86]

(Table 1) contd.....

Sl. No	Protein	Functions	Findings in DR	Inference	Ref.
3	Pigment epithelium derived factor (PEDF)	Maintenance of vascular permeability and angiogenesis; required for the stability of neurons	Decreased expression of PEDF along with increased expression of VEGF	Reciprocal regulation of PEDF and VEGF is essential to maintain retinal homeostasis	[89]
4	C3, C1	Plays a role in maintain innate immune system and activation of microglia in the retina	Increased expression	Activation of complement pathway	[87]
5	Cadherin-5	Maintenance of endothelial cell (EC)barrier	Reduced level in DR eye	Reduction of cadherin expression cause increased vascular leakage	[93]
6	MCP1	Regulate infiltration and migration of monocytes; activation of microglia	Increased expression after 4 weeks of diabetes	Neuronal MCP 1 induced microglial activation.	[88]
7	Synaptophysin	Synaptic vesicle protein	Down regulation of synaptophysin	Neuronal dysfunction	[94, 95]
8	Carbonic anhydrase	For the conversion of CO_2 and water in to carbonic acid	Increased expression in the vitreous of DR subjects	Promote retinal vessel leakage by activating intrinsic coagulation pathway, neurovascular edema	[87, 96]

CONCLUDING REMARKS

The current therapeutic strategies like laser photocoagulation, anti-VEGF therapy, and vitreous surgery are mainly focused on the microvasculature complications of the retina. However, neurodegeneration is one of the major causes of vision impairment in DR. Despite being considered a metabolic disorder, DR is an inflammatory disorder of the CNS. Retinal homeostasis is maintained by the glial cells. Many of the reasons for neuronal damage and vascular changes in the DR are associated with glial activation, including gliosis, altered metabolism, VEGF production as well as glutamate excitotoxicity. The major point of concern in DR is the glial activation and associated release of various cytokines, which induce the progression of the disease. The increased secretion of inflammatory cytokines in the retina and the altered metabolism cause severe damage to the neurons. These neurodegenerative changes precede the vascular damage in DR. Identification of the neural changes might help in early prediction and effective prevention of the disease. Targeting glial activation and associated changes like inflammation in the DR may give a better understanding and management strategies for DR.

CONFLICT OF INTEREST

The author (editor) declares no conflict of interest, financial or otherwise.

ACKNOWLEDGEMENTS

Supported in parts by a grant from the Centre for Excellence (COE) grant (on Diabetic Retinopathy by Department of Biotechnology, Government of India and Hyderabad Eye Research foundation to IK.

REFERENCES

[1]   Gorman AM. Neuronal cell death in neurodegenerative diseases: recurring themes around protein handling. J Cell Mol Med 2008; 12(6A): 2263-80.
[http://dx.doi.org/10.1111/j.1582-4934.2008.00402.x] [PMID: 18624755]

[2]   Brahmachari S, Fung YK, Pahan K. Induction of glial fibrillary acidic protein expression in astrocytes by nitric oxide. J Neurosci 2006; 26(18): 4930-9.
[http://dx.doi.org/10.1523/JNEUROSCI.5480-05.2006] [PMID: 16672668]

[3]   Lull ME, Block ML. Microglial activation and chronic neurodegeneration. Neurotherapeutics 2010; 7(4): 354-65.
[http://dx.doi.org/10.1016/j.nurt.2010.05.014] [PMID: 20880500]

[4]   Goedert M. NEURODEGENERATION. Alzheimer's and Parkinson's diseases: The prion concept in relation to assembled Aβ, tau, and α-synuclein. Science 2015; 349(6248): 1255555.
[http://dx.doi.org/10.1126/science.1255555] [PMID: 26250687]

[5]   Gil JM, Rego AC. Mechanisms of neurodegeneration in Huntington's disease. Eur J Neurosci 2008; 27(11): 2803-20.
[http://dx.doi.org/10.1111/j.1460-9568.2008.06310.x] [PMID: 18588526]

[6]   Crish SD, Calkins DJ. Neurodegeneration in glaucoma: progression and calcium-dependent intracellular mechanisms. Neuroscience 2011; 176: 1-11.
[http://dx.doi.org/10.1016/j.neuroscience.2010.12.036] [PMID: 21187126]

[7]   Koch SF, Tsai YT, Duong JK, *et al.* Halting progressive neurodegeneration in advanced retinitis pigmentosa. J Clin Invest 2015; 125(9): 3704-13.
[http://dx.doi.org/10.1172/JCI82462] [PMID: 26301813]

[8]   Kaarniranta K, Salminen A, Haapasalo A, Soininen H, Hiltunen M. Age-related macular degeneration (AMD): Alzheimer's disease in the eye? J Alzheimers Dis 2011; 24(4): 615-31.
[PMID: 21297256]

[9]   Barber AJ. A new view of diabetic retinopathy: a neurodegenerative disease of the eye. Prog Neuropsychopharmacol Biol Psychiatry 2003; 27(2): 283-90.
[http://dx.doi.org/10.1016/S0278-5846(03)00023-X] [PMID: 12657367]

[10]   Gardner TW, Antonetti DA, Barber AJ, LaNoue KF, Levison SW. Diabetic retinopathy: more than meets the eye. Surv Ophthalmol 2002; 47 (Suppl. 2): S253-62.
[http://dx.doi.org/10.1016/S0039-6257(02)00387-9] [PMID: 12507627]

[11]   Yau JW, Rogers SL, Kawasaki R, *et al.* Global prevalence and major risk factors of diabetic retinopathy. Diabetes Care 2012; 35(3): 556-64.
[http://dx.doi.org/10.2337/dc11-1909] [PMID: 22301125]

[12] Klein R. The epidemiology of diabetic retinopathy: findings from the Wisconsin Epidemiologic Study of Diabetic Retinopathy. Int Ophthalmol Clin 1987; 27(4): 230-8.
[http://dx.doi.org/10.1097/00004397-198702740-00003] [PMID: 3319933]

[13] Klein R, Klein BE, Moss SE, Davis MD, DeMets DL. The Wisconsin epidemiologic study of diabetic retinopathy. II. Prevalence and risk of diabetic retinopathy when age at diagnosis is less than 30 years. Arch Ophthalmol 1984; 102(4): 520-6.
[http://dx.doi.org/10.1001/archopht.1984.01040030398010] [PMID: 6367724]

[14] Wild S, Roglic G, Green A, Sicree R, King H. Global prevalence of diabetes: estimates for the year 2000 and projections for 2030. Diabetes Care 2004; 27(5): 1047-53.
[http://dx.doi.org/10.2337/diacare.27.5.1047] [PMID: 15111519]

[15] Krishnaiah S, Das T, Nirmalan PK, *et al.* Risk factors for diabetic retinopathy: Findings from The Andhra Pradesh Eye Disease Study. Clin Ophthalmol 2007; 1(4): 475-82.
[PMID: 19668525]

[16] Viswanath K, McGavin DD. Diabetic retinopathy: clinical findings and management. Community Eye Health 2003; 16(46): 21-4.
[PMID: 17491851]

[17] Caldwell RB, Bartoli M, Behzadian MA, *et al.* Vascular endothelial growth factor and diabetic retinopathy: role of oxidative stress. Curr Drug Targets 2005; 6(4): 511-24.
[http://dx.doi.org/10.2174/1389450054021981] [PMID: 16026270]

[18] Olmos LC, Lee RK. Medical and surgical treatment of neovascular glaucoma. Int Ophthalmol Clin 2011; 51(3): 27-36.
[http://dx.doi.org/10.1097/IIO.0b013e31821e5960] [PMID: 21633236]

[19] Ferris FL III, Patz A. Macular edema. A complication of diabetic retinopathy. Surv Ophthalmol 1984; 28 (Suppl.): 452-61.
[http://dx.doi.org/10.1016/0039-6257(84)90227-3] [PMID: 6379946]

[20] Park YG, Roh YJ. New Diagnostic and Therapeutic Approaches for Preventing the Progression of Diabetic Retinopathy. J Diabetes Res 2016; 2016: 1753584.

[21] Hombrebueno JR, Ali IH, Xu H, Chen M. Sustained intraocular VEGF neutralization results in retinal neurodegeneration in the Ins2(Akita) diabetic mouse. Sci Rep 2015; 5: 18316.
[http://dx.doi.org/10.1038/srep18316] [PMID: 26671074]

[22] Perron M, Harris WA. Determination of vertebrate retinal progenitor cell fate by the Notch pathway and basic helix-loop-helix transcription factors. Cell Mol Life Sci 2000; 57(2): 215-23.
[http://dx.doi.org/10.1007/PL00000685] [PMID: 10766018]

[23] Shin ES, Sorenson CM, Sheibani N. Diabetes and retinal vascular dysfunction. J Ophthalmic Vis Res 2014; 9(3): 362-73.
[PMID: 25667739]

[24] Verrotti A, Lobefalo L, Petitti MT, *et al.* Relationship between contrast sensitivity and metabolic control in diabetics with and without retinopathy. Ann Med 1998; 30(4): 369-74.
[http://dx.doi.org/10.3109/07853899809029936] [PMID: 9783835]

[25] Tregear SJ, Knowles PJ, Ripley LG, Casswell AG. Chromatic-contrast threshold impairment in diabetes. Eye (Lond) 1997; 11(Pt 4): 537-46.
[http://dx.doi.org/10.1038/eye.1997.140] [PMID: 9425421]

[26] Daley ML, Watzke RC, Riddle MC. Early loss of blue-sensitive color vision in patients with type I diabetes. Diabetes Care 1987; 10(6): 777-81.
[http://dx.doi.org/10.2337/diacare.10.6.777] [PMID: 3501362]

[27] Sokol S, Moskowitz A, Skarf B, Evans R, Molitch M, Senior B. Contrast sensitivity in diabetics with and without background retinopathy. Arch Ophthalmol 1985; 103(1): 51-4.

[http://dx.doi.org/10.1001/archopht.1985.01050010055018] [PMID: 3977675]

[28]   Ng DS, Chiang PP, Tan G, *et al*. Retinal ganglion cell neuronal damage in diabetes and diabetic retinopathy. Clin Experiment Ophthalmol 2016; 44(4): 243-50.
[http://dx.doi.org/10.1111/ceo.12724] [PMID: 26872562]

[29]   Verma A, Raman R, Vaitheeswaran K, *et al*. Does neuronal damage precede vascular damage in subjects with type 2 diabetes mellitus and having no clinical diabetic retinopathy? Ophthalmic Res 2012; 47(4): 202-7.
[http://dx.doi.org/10.1159/000333220] [PMID: 22179629]

[30]   Bonnin S, Tadayoni R, Erginay A, Massin P, Dupas B. Correlation between ganglion cell layer thinning and poor visual function after resolution of diabetic macular edema. Invest Ophthalmol Vis Sci 2015; 56(2): 978-82.
[http://dx.doi.org/10.1167/iovs.14-15503] [PMID: 25574055]

[31]   Chhablani J, Sharma A, Goud A, *et al*. Neurodegeneration in type 2 diabetes: evidence from spectral-domain optical coherence tomography. Invest Ophthalmol Vis Sci 2015; 56(11): 6333-8.
[http://dx.doi.org/10.1167/iovs.15-17334] [PMID: 26436886]

[32]   Kern TS, Barber AJ. Retinal ganglion cells in diabetes. J Physiol 2008; 586(18): 4401-8.
[http://dx.doi.org/10.1113/jphysiol.2008.156695] [PMID: 18565995]

[33]   Barber AJ, Lieth E, Khin SA, Antonetti DA, Buchanan AG, Gardner TW. Neural apoptosis in the retina during experimental and human diabetes. Early onset and effect of insulin. J Clin Invest 1998; 102(4): 783-91.
[http://dx.doi.org/10.1172/JCI2425] [PMID: 9710447]

[34]   Barber AJ, Antonetti DA, Kern TS, *et al*. The Ins2Akita mouse as a model of early retinal complications in diabetes. Invest Ophthalmol Vis Sci 2005; 46(6): 2210-8.
[http://dx.doi.org/10.1167/iovs.04-1340] [PMID: 15914643]

[35]   Djamgoz MB, Hankins MW, Hirano J, Archer SN. Neurobiology of retinal dopamine in relation to degenerative states of the tissue. Vision Res 1997; 37(24): 3509-29.
[http://dx.doi.org/10.1016/S0042-6989(97)00129-6] [PMID: 9425527]

[36]   Amthor FR, Keyser KT, Dmitrieva NA. Effects of the destruction of starburst-cholinergic amacrine cells by the toxin AF64A on rabbit retinal directional selectivity. Vis Neurosci 2002; 19(4): 495-509.
[http://dx.doi.org/10.1017/S0952523802194119] [PMID: 12511082]

[37]   Gastinger MJ, Singh RS, Barber AJ. Loss of cholinergic and dopaminergic amacrine cells in streptozotocin-diabetic rat and Ins2Akita-diabetic mouse retinas. Invest Ophthalmol Vis Sci 2006; 47(7): 3143-50.
[http://dx.doi.org/10.1167/iovs.05-1376] [PMID: 16799061]

[38]   Yang Q, Xu Y, Xie P, Cheng H, Song Q, Su T, *et al*. Retinal Neurodegeneration in db/db Mice at the Early Period of Diabetes. J Ophthalmol 2015; 2015: 757412.

[39]   Bek T. Immunohistochemical characterization of retinal glial cell changes in areas of vascular occlusion secondary to diabetic retinopathy. Acta Ophthalmol Scand 1997; 75(4): 388-92.
[http://dx.doi.org/10.1111/j.1600-0420.1997.tb00395.x] [PMID: 9374245]

[40]   Mizutani M, Gerhardinger C, Lorenzi M. Müller cell changes in human diabetic retinopathy. Diabetes 1998; 47(3): 445-9.
[http://dx.doi.org/10.2337/diabetes.47.3.445] [PMID: 9519752]

[41]   Qin Y, Xu G, Wang W. Dendritic abnormalities in retinal ganglion cells of three-month diabetic rats. Curr Eye Res 2006; 31(11): 967-74.
[http://dx.doi.org/10.1080/02713680600987674] [PMID: 17114122]

[42]   Martin PM, Roon P, Van Ells TK, Ganapathy V, Smith SB. Death of retinal neurons in streptozotocin-induced diabetic mice. Invest Ophthalmol Vis Sci 2004; 45(9): 3330-6.
[http://dx.doi.org/10.1167/iovs.04-0247] [PMID: 15326158]

[43]   Abu-El-Asrar AM, Dralands L, Missotten L, Al-Jadaan IA, Geboes K. Expression of apoptosis markers in the retinas of human subjects with diabetes. Invest Ophthalmol Vis Sci 2004; 45(8): 2760-6.
[http://dx.doi.org/10.1167/iovs.03-1392] [PMID: 15277502]

[44]   Valverde AM, Miranda S, García-Ramírez M, González-Rodriguez Á, Hernández C, Simó R. Proapoptotic and survival signaling in the neuroretina at early stages of diabetic retinopathy. Mol Vis 2013; 19: 47-53.
[PMID: 23335850]

[45]   Park SH, Park JW, Park SJ, *et al.* Apoptotic death of photoreceptors in the streptozotocin-induced diabetic rat retina. Diabetologia 2003; 46(9): 1260-8.
[http://dx.doi.org/10.1007/s00125-003-1177-6] [PMID: 12898017]

[46]   Simó R, Carrasco E, García-Ramírez M, Hernández C. Angiogenic and antiangiogenic factors in proliferative diabetic retinopathy. Curr Diabetes Rev 2006; 2(1): 71-98.
[http://dx.doi.org/10.2174/157339906775473671] [PMID: 18220619]

[47]   Carrasco E, Hernández C, Miralles A, Huguet P, Farrés J, Simó R. Lower somatostatin expression is an early event in diabetic retinopathy and is associated with retinal neurodegeneration. Diabetes Care 2007; 30(11): 2902-8.
[http://dx.doi.org/10.2337/dc07-0332] [PMID: 17704349]

[48]   Piano I, Novelli E, Della Santina L, Strettoi E, Cervetto L, Gargini C. Involvement of autophagic pathway in the progression of retinal degeneration in a mouse model of diabetes. Front Cell Neurosci 2016; 10: 42.
[http://dx.doi.org/10.3389/fncel.2016.00042] [PMID: 26924963]

[49]   Joussen AM, Poulaki V, Le ML, *et al.* A central role for inflammation in the pathogenesis of diabetic retinopathy. FASEB J 2004; 18(12): 1450-2.
[PMID: 15231732]

[50]   Demircan N, Safran BG, Soylu M, Ozcan AA, Sizmaz S. Determination of vitreous interleukin-1 (IL-1) and tumour necrosis factor (TNF) levels in proliferative diabetic retinopathy. Eye (Lond) 2006; 20(12): 1366-9.
[http://dx.doi.org/10.1038/sj.eye.6702138] [PMID: 16284605]

[51]   Abu el Asrar AM, Maimone D, Morse PH, Gregory S, Reder AT. Cytokines in the vitreous of patients with proliferative diabetic retinopathy. Am J Ophthalmol 1992; 114(6): 731-6.
[http://dx.doi.org/10.1016/S0002-9394(14)74052-8] [PMID: 1463043]

[52]   Querques G, Delle Noci N. Proinflammatory cytokines and angiogenic and antiangiogenic factors in vitreous of patients with proliferative diabetic retinopathy and Eales' disease (ED). Retina 2009; 29(1): 121-3.
[http://dx.doi.org/10.1097/IAE.0b013e31818baa03] [PMID: 18936719]

[53]   Garland DL, Fernandez-Godino R, Kaur I, *et al.* Mouse genetics and proteomic analyses demonstrate a critical role for complement in a model of DHRD/ML, an inherited macular degeneration. Hum Mol Genet 2014; 23(1): 52-68.
[http://dx.doi.org/10.1093/hmg/ddt395] [PMID: 23943789]

[54]   Członkowska A, Kurkowska-Jastrzębska I. Inflammation and gliosis in neurological diseases--clinical implications. J Neuroimmunol 2011; 231(1-2): 78-85.
[http://dx.doi.org/10.1016/j.jneuroim.2010.09.020] [PMID: 20943275]

[55]   Feng Y, Wang Y, Stock O, *et al.* Vasoregression linked to neuronal damage in the rat with defect of polycystin-2. PLoS One 2009; 4(10): e7328.
[http://dx.doi.org/10.1371/journal.pone.0007328] [PMID: 19806208]

[56]   Rosa JM, Bos R, Sack GS, *et al.* Neuron-glia signaling in developing retina mediated by neurotransmitter spillover. eLife 2015; 4: 4.

[http://dx.doi.org/10.7554/eLife.09590] [PMID: 26274565]

[57]   Innocenti B, Parpura V, Haydon PG. Imaging extracellular waves of glutamate during calcium signaling in cultured astrocytes. J Neurosci 2000; 20(5): 1800-8.
[PMID: 10684881]

[58]   Gerhardinger C, Costa MB, Coulombe MC, Toth I, Hoehn T, Grosu P. Expression of acute-phase response proteins in retinal Müller cells in diabetes. Invest Ophthalmol Vis Sci 2005; 46(1): 349-57.
[http://dx.doi.org/10.1167/iovs.04-0860] [PMID: 15623795]

[59]   Yego EC, Vincent JA, Sarthy V, Busik JV, Mohr S. Differential regulation of high glucose-induced glyceraldehyde-3-phosphate dehydrogenase nuclear accumulation in Müller cells by IL-1beta and IL-6. Invest Ophthalmol Vis Sci 2009; 50(4): 1920-8.
[http://dx.doi.org/10.1167/iovs.08-2082] [PMID: 19060282]

[60]   Newman E, Reichenbach A. The Müller cell: a functional element of the retina. Trends Neurosci 1996; 19(8): 307-12.
[http://dx.doi.org/10.1016/0166-2236(96)10040-0] [PMID: 8843598]

[61]   Li Q, Puro DG. Diabetes-induced dysfunction of the glutamate transporter in retinal Müller cells. Invest Ophthalmol Vis Sci 2002; 43(9): 3109-16.
[PMID: 12202536]

[62]   Azuma N, Kawamura M, Kohsaka S. Morphological and immunohistochemical studies on degenerative changes of the retina and the optic nerve in neonatal rats injected with monosodium-L-glutamate. Nippon Ganka Gakkai Zasshi 1989; 93(1): 72-9.
[PMID: 2750602]

[63]   Lieth E, Barber AJ, Xu B, *et al.* Glial reactivity and impaired glutamate metabolism in short-term experimental diabetic retinopathy. Diabetes 1998; 47(5): 815-20.
[http://dx.doi.org/10.2337/diabetes.47.5.815] [PMID: 9588455]

[64]   Derouiche A, Rauen T. Coincidence of L-glutamate/L-aspartate transporter (GLAST) and glutamine synthetase (GS) immunoreactions in retinal glia: evidence for coupling of GLAST and GS in transmitter clearance. J Neurosci Res 1995; 42(1): 131-43.
[http://dx.doi.org/10.1002/jnr.490420115] [PMID: 8531222]

[65]   Lieth E, LaNoue KF, Antonetti DA, Ratz M. Diabetes reduces glutamate oxidation and glutamine synthesis in the retina. Exp Eye Res 2000; 70(6): 723-30.
[http://dx.doi.org/10.1006/exer.2000.0840] [PMID: 10843776]

[66]   Dheen ST, Kaur C, Ling EA. Microglial activation and its implications in the brain diseases. Curr Med Chem 2007; 14(11): 1189-97.
[http://dx.doi.org/10.2174/092986707780597961] [PMID: 17504139]

[67]   Krady JK, Basu A, Allen CM, *et al.* Minocycline reduces proinflammatory cytokine expression, microglial activation, and caspase-3 activation in a rodent model of diabetic retinopathy. Diabetes 2005; 54(5): 1559-65.
[http://dx.doi.org/10.2337/diabetes.54.5.1559] [PMID: 15855346]

[68]   Grigsby JG, Cardona SM, Pouw CE, Muniz A, Mendiola AS, Tsin AT, *et al.* The role of microglia in diabetic retinopathy. J Ophthalmol 2014; 2014: 705783.

[69]   Zeng HY, Green WR, Tso MO. Microglial activation in human diabetic retinopathy. Arch Ophthalmol 2008; 126(2): 227-32.
[http://dx.doi.org/10.1001/archophthalmol.2007.65] [PMID: 18268214]

[70]   Omri S, Behar-Cohen F, de Kozak Y, *et al.* Microglia/macrophages migrate through retinal epithelium barrier by a transcellular route in diabetic retinopathy: role of PKCζ in the Goto Kakizaki rat model. Am J Pathol 2011; 179(2): 942-53.
[http://dx.doi.org/10.1016/j.ajpath.2011.04.018] [PMID: 21712024]

[71]   Ibrahim AS, El-Remessy AB, Matragoon S, *et al.* Retinal microglial activation and inflammation

induced by amadori-glycated albumin in a rat model of diabetes. Diabetes 2011; 60(4): 1122-33.
[http://dx.doi.org/10.2337/db10-1160] [PMID: 21317295]

[72] Cardona SM, Mendiola AS, Yang YC, Adkins SL, Torres V, Cardona AE. Disruption of Fractalkine
       Signaling Leads to Microglial Activation and Neuronal Damage in the Diabetic Retina. ASN Neuro
       2015; 7(5): 1759091415608204.
       [http://dx.doi.org/10.1177/1759091415608204] [PMID: 26514658]

[73] Kowluru RA, Abbas SN. Diabetes-induced mitochondrial dysfunction in the retina. Invest Ophthalmol
       Vis Sci 2003; 44(12): 5327-34.
       [http://dx.doi.org/10.1167/iovs.03-0353] [PMID: 14638734]

[74] Silva KC, Rosales MA, Biswas SK, Lopes de Faria JB, Lopes de Faria JM. Diabetic retinal
       neurodegeneration is associated with mitochondrial oxidative stress and is improved by an angiotensin
       receptor blocker in a model combining hypertension and diabetes. Diabetes 2009; 58(6): 1382-90.
       [http://dx.doi.org/10.2337/db09-0166] [PMID: 19289456]

[75] Cimini S, Rizzardini M, Biella G, Cantoni L. Hypoxia causes autophagic stress and derangement of
       metabolic adaptation in a cell model of amyotrophic lateral sclerosis. J Neurochem 2014; 129(3): 413-
       25.
       [http://dx.doi.org/10.1111/jnc.12642] [PMID: 24359187]

[76] Lin WJ, Kuang HY. Oxidative stress induces autophagy in response to multiple noxious stimuli in
       retinal ganglion cells. Autophagy 2014; 10(10): 1692-701.
       [http://dx.doi.org/10.4161/auto.36076] [PMID: 25207555]

[77] Schmidt KG, Bergert H, Funk RH. Neurodegenerative diseases of the retina and potential for
       protection and recovery. Curr Neuropharmacol 2008; 6(2): 164-78.
       [http://dx.doi.org/10.2174/157015908784533851] [PMID: 19305795]

[78] Wang J, Xu X, Elliott MH, Zhu M, Le YZ. Müller cell-derived VEGF is essential for diabetes-induced
       retinal inflammation and vascular leakage. Diabetes 2010; 59(9): 2297-305.
       [http://dx.doi.org/10.2337/db09-1420] [PMID: 20530741]

[79] Bai Y, Ma JX, Guo J, *et al.* Müller cell-derived VEGF is a significant contributor to retinal
       neovascularization. J Pathol 2009; 219(4): 446-54.
       [http://dx.doi.org/10.1002/path.2611] [PMID: 19768732]

[80] Heesom AE, Hibberd ML, Millward A, Demaine AG. Polymorphism in the 5'-end of the aldose
       reductase gene is strongly associated with the development of diabetic nephropathy in type I diabetes.
       Diabetes 1997; 46(2): 287-91.
       [http://dx.doi.org/10.2337/diab.46.2.287] [PMID: 9000706]

[81] Asnaghi V, Gerhardinger C, Hoehn T, Adeboje A, Lorenzi M. A role for the polyol pathway in the
       early neuroretinal apoptosis and glial changes induced by diabetes in the rat. Diabetes 2003; 52(2):
       506-11.
       [http://dx.doi.org/10.2337/diabetes.52.2.506] [PMID: 12540628]

[82] Al-Kateb H, Mirea L, Xie X, *et al.* Multiple variants in vascular endothelial growth factor (VEGFA)
       are risk factors for time to severe retinopathy in type 1 diabetes: the DCCT/EDIC genetics study.
       Diabetes 2007; 56(8): 2161-8.
       [http://dx.doi.org/10.2337/db07-0376] [PMID: 17513698]

[83] Brucklacher RM, Patel KM, VanGuilder HD, *et al.* Whole genome assessment of the retinal response
       to diabetes reveals a progressive neurovascular inflammatory response. BMC Med Genomics 2008; 1:
       26.
       [http://dx.doi.org/10.1186/1755-8794-1-26] [PMID: 18554398]

[84] Lin PT, Gleeson JG, Corbo JC, Flanagan L, Walsh CA. DCAMKL1 encodes a protein kinase with
       homology to doublecortin that regulates microtubule polymerization. J Neurosci 2000; 20(24): 9152-
       61.
       [PMID: 11124993]

[85]   Berger UV, Hediger MA. Distribution of peptide transporter PEPT2 mRNA in the rat nervous system. Anat Embryol (Berl) 1999; 199(5): 439-49.
[http://dx.doi.org/10.1007/s004290050242] [PMID: 10221455]

[86]   Fort PE, Freeman WM, Losiewicz MK, Singh RS, Gardner TW. The retinal proteome in experimental diabetic retinopathy: up-regulation of crystallins and reversal by systemic and periocular insulin. Mol Cell Proteomics 2009; 8(4): 767-79.
[http://dx.doi.org/10.1074/mcp.M800326-MCP200] [PMID: 19049959]

[87]   Gao BB, Chen X, Timothy N, Aiello LP, Feener EP. Characterization of the vitreous proteome in diabetes without diabetic retinopathy and diabetes with proliferative diabetic retinopathy. J Proteome Res 2008; 7(6): 2516-25.
[http://dx.doi.org/10.1021/pr800112g] [PMID: 18433156]

[88]   Dong N, Li X, Xiao L, Yu W, Wang B, Chu L. Upregulation of retinal neuronal MCP-1 in the rodent model of diabetic retinopathy and its function *in vitro*. Invest Ophthalmol Vis Sci 2012; 53(12): 7567-75.
[http://dx.doi.org/10.1167/iovs.12-9446] [PMID: 23010641]

[89]   Zhang SX, Wang JJ, Gao G, Parke K, Ma JX. Pigment epithelium-derived factor downregulates vascular endothelial growth factor (VEGF) expression and inhibits VEGF-VEGF receptor 2 binding in diabetic retinopathy. J Mol Endocrinol 2006; 37(1): 1-12.
[http://dx.doi.org/10.1677/jme.1.02008] [PMID: 16901919]

[90]   Sinha D, Klise A, Sergeev Y, *et al.* betaA3/A1-crystallin in astroglial cells regulates retinal vascular remodeling during development. Mol Cell Neurosci 2008; 37(1): 85-95.
[http://dx.doi.org/10.1016/j.mcn.2007.08.016] [PMID: 17931883]

[91]   Luo C, Chen M, Xu H. Complement gene expression and regulation in mouse retina and retinal pigment epithelium/choroid. Mol Vis 2011; 17: 1588-97.
[PMID: 21738388]

[92]   Cheng L, Bu H, Portillo JA, *et al.* Modulation of retinal Müller cells by complement receptor C5aR. Invest Ophthalmol Vis Sci 2013; 54(13): 8191-8.
[http://dx.doi.org/10.1167/iovs.13-12428] [PMID: 24265019]

[93]   Davidson MK, Russ PK, Glick GG, Hoffman LH, Chang MS, Haselton FR. Reduced expression of the adherens junction protein cadherin-5 in a diabetic retina. Am J Ophthalmol 2000; 129(2): 267-9.
[http://dx.doi.org/10.1016/S0002-9394(99)00323-2] [PMID: 10682990]

[94]   Kurihara T, Ozawa Y, Nagai N, *et al.* Angiotensin II type 1 receptor signaling contributes to synaptophysin degradation and neuronal dysfunction in the diabetic retina. Diabetes 2008; 57(8): 2191-8.
[http://dx.doi.org/10.2337/db07-1281] [PMID: 18487452]

[95]   VanGuilder HD, Brucklacher RM, Patel K, Ellis RW, Freeman WM, Barber AJ. Diabetes downregulates presynaptic proteins and reduces basal synapsin I phosphorylation in rat retina. Eur J Neurosci 2008; 28(1): 1-11.
[http://dx.doi.org/10.1111/j.1460-9568.2008.06322.x] [PMID: 18662330]

[96]   Gao BB, Clermont A, Rook S, *et al.* Extracellular carbonic anhydrase mediates hemorrhagic retinal and cerebral vascular permeability through prekallikrein activation. Nat Med 2007; 13(2): 181-8.
[http://dx.doi.org/10.1038/nm1534] [PMID: 17259996]

CHAPTER 5

Rhodopsin Traffics to the Rod Outer Segment in the Absence of Homodimeric and Heterotrimeric Kinesin-2

Li Jiang, Jeanne M. Frederick and **Wolfgang Baehr**[*]

Department of Ophthalmology and Visual Sciences, University of Utah Health Science Center, Salt Lake City, UT 84132, USA

Abstract: Homodimeric (KIF17) and heterotrimeric kinesin-2 (KIF3A, KIF3B and KAP) molecular motors are essential for anterograde intraflagellar transport (IFT) among invertebrates. Here we show that deletion of KIF3A in embryonic mouse retina interferes with IFT by preventing transition zone and axoneme formation. Absence of outer segments leads to severe mistrafficking of rhodopsin and rapid degeneration. By contrast, deletion of KIF3A in the adult mouse by tamoxifen-induction reveals normal rhodopsin transport to outer segments with failure of outer segment (OS) maintenance. Germline deletion of KIF17, a motor that cooperates with heterotrimeric kinesin-2 among invertebrates, affected neither OS structure nor photoreceptor morphology/ function thereby excluding an essential role of KIF17 in photoreceptor IFT. A KIF3A/KIF17 double knockout phenocopies a rod-specific KIF3A knockout. We conclude IFT is not required for rhodopsin transport to the OS but rather, anterograde IFT mediated by KIF3 participates in photoreceptor transition zone (PTZ) and axoneme formation.

Keywords: Anterograde intraflagellar transport (IFT), Conditional knockouts, Heterotrimeric kinesin-2, Homodimeric kinesin-2, Mouse photoreceptors, Rhodopsin trafficking.

INTRODUCTION

The light-sensitive photoreceptor sensory cilium, regarded as a modified primary cilium, is comprised of OS disc membranes, a basal body (microtubule-organizing center) and an axoneme. Each OS communicates with its inner segment (IS) through a connecting cilium which is a structure equivalent to the transition zone of primary cilia [1]. OS proteins, synthesized in the IS, must traffic through the photoreceptor transition zone (PTZ) to be incorporated into nascent discs. Intra-

---

[*] **Corresponding author Wolfgang Baehr:** Moran Eye Center, University of Utah Health Science Center, Salt Lake City, UT 84132, USA; Tel: 801-585-6643; E-mail: wbaehr@hsc.utah.edu

flagellar transport (IFT), a bidirectional ciliary trafficking pathway conserved among invertebrates and vertebrates [2], has been suggested to traffic rhodopsin and other OS proteins together with IFT particles (IFT-A and IFT-B) along the ciliary axoneme [3, 4].

Heterotrimeric kinesin-2 (KIF3, consisting of KIF3A, KIF3B and KAP subunits) [5] and homodimeric kinesin-2 (KIF17) [6] are canonical anterograde IFT motors present in a broad range of species [7 - 9]. KIF17 and KIF3 are thought to cooperate during ciliogenesis in which KIF3 builds the axoneme core and KIF17 the axoneme distal segments (Fig. **1**) [10, 11]. However, interaction of KIF17 with KIF3, and KIF17 contribution to vertebrate ciliogenesis or membrane protein trafficking are unclear. Disruption of KIF3A, the obligatory subunit of KIF3, caused rapid photoreceptor degeneration and OS protein mistrafficking [12, 13]. However, we showed that rod-specific knockout of KIF3A did not prevent trafficking of rhodopsin to the OS even as the OS degenerated [14]. A second anterograde motor candidate in photoreceptors is KIF17, which mediates IFT in *C. elegans* (Osm-3) [11] and was suggested to participate in zebrafish photoreceptor development [15].

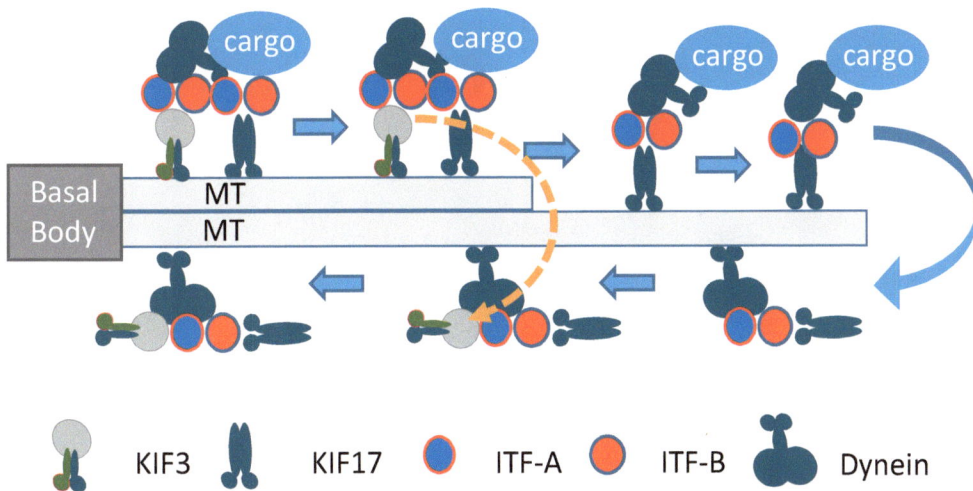

Fig. (1). Intraflagellar transport. KIF3 and KIF17 cooperate in anterograde transport of cargo at the proximal axoneme (MT doublet). Cargo consists of IFT particles, dynein motors, axoneme building blocks and axoneme stabilizing factors. Whereas KIF3 turns around, KIF17 continues to move cargo distally along the MT singlet. Retrograde transport is powered by dynein motors.

This study explores the roles of KIF3 and KIF17 in mouse photoreceptor ciliogenesis and rhodopsin trafficking. We deleted KIF3A in retina during embryonic photoreceptor development and in the adult mouse with tamoxifen-induction. Retina-specific deletion of KIF3A during early development resulted in failure to form PTZs and OSs. Depletion of KIF3A in adult photoreceptors by tamoxifen-induction resulted in progressive shortening of the OS axoneme despite continued rhodopsin trafficking. Germline deletion of KIF17 did not produce a recognizable retina phenotype up to the age of one year. Our data indicate that KIF3-driven IFT functions primarily in photoreceptor ciliogenesis and axoneme stabilization rather than rhodopsin transport.

Ubiquitous Expression of KIF3A and KIF17

KIF3A and KIF17 are expressed in most mouse tissues, prominently in testes, ovary, lung, brain and thymus, and both are present in the eye (Fig. **2A**). In mouse retina, KIF3A (Fig. **2B**) and KIF17 (Fig. **2C**) are observed abundantly in photoreceptor inner segments (IS) and the outer nuclear layer (ONL).

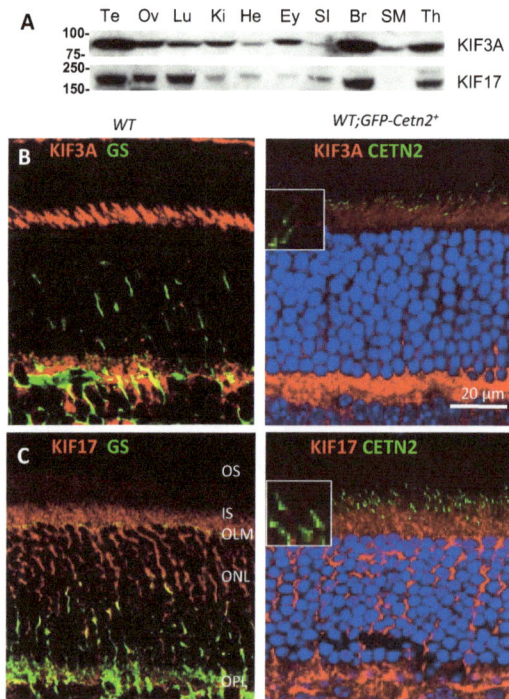

Fig. (2). KIF3A and KIF17 expressions in retina. (A) Multiple tissue immunoblot probed with anti-KIF3A (upper panel) and anti-KIF17 (bottom panel) antibodies, respectively. **(B)** KIF3A in WT (left) and *GFP-Cetn2+* (right) mouse retinas at one month of age. Centrin 2 (CETN2) is a calmodulin-like Ca^{2+}-binding protein associated with centrioles and transition zones. Left, colabeling of anti-KIF3A (red) with anti-glutamine synthase (GS, a Muller cell marker, green). Right inset, enlargement of GFP-CETN2-labeled basal bodies and connecting cilia (PTZ). **(C)** KIF17 (red) expression in WT (left) and *GFP-Cetn2+* (right) mouse retinas. KIF17 label overlaps with GS at ONL in Muller glia, but not with basal bodies (inset). Right inset, basal bodies and transition zones identified by GFP-CETN2. OS, outer segment; IS, inner segment; OLM, outer limiting membrane; ONL, outer nuclear layer; OPL, outer plexiform layer.

KIF3A was also found prominently at the outer plexiform layer (OPL) where photoreceptor synaptic terminals contact the dendrites of bipolar and horizontal cells. Colabeling with antibody directed against glutamine synthetase (GS), a Müller cell marker, demonstrates that KIF17 is also expressed in Müller cell processes of the ONL (Fig. **2C**, left). Centrin 2 (CETN2), a centriole and PTZ marker, was used to delineate expression of KIF3A and KIF17 at the basal body. In transgenic mice expressing GFP-CETN2, KIF3A localized at the IS and proximal OS axoneme (Fig. **2B**, right, inset).

Early Loss of KIF3A Arrests Ciliogenesis

We deleted KIF3A conditionally in photoreceptor progenitors by mating *Kif3a* floxed mice [12, 14] with Six3Cre mice [16] to generate *Kif3a^{f/f};Six3Cre^{+}* (abbreviated as *^{emb}Kif3a^{-/-}*) (Fig. **3A**). KIF3A is expected to be deleted before photoreceptor differentiation in the *^{emb}Kif3a^{-/-}* mouse. The *^{emb}Kif3a^{-/-}* retina developed normal outer nuclear layer (ONL) lamination through P10 (Fig. **3B**), but began to degenerate at P10-11. Degeneration was nearly complete at P24.

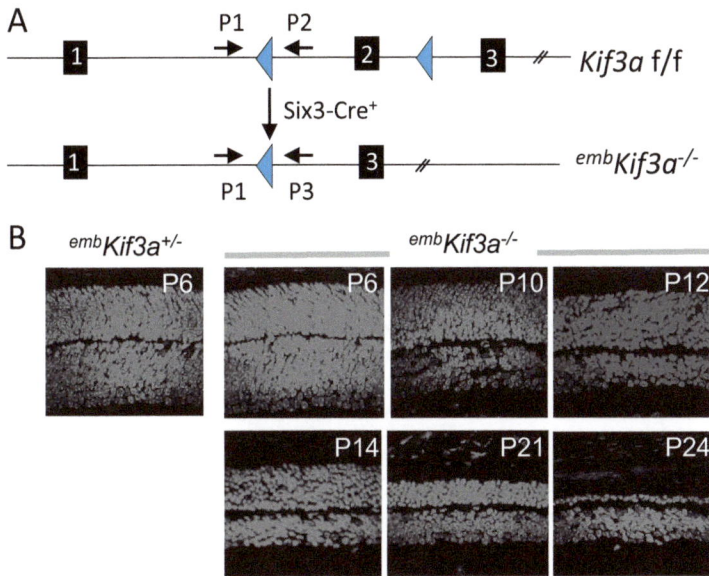

Fig. (3). Generation of embryonic retina-specific Kif3a knockouts. (A) *Kif3a^{f/f}* mice were mated with Six3*Cre* mice to generate *^{emb}Kif3a^{-/-}* mice in which exon 2 is deleted. **(B)** Retina transverse sections at various postnatal times. ONL degeneration begins at P12, and only cone nuclei remain at P24.

KIF3A localized to the inner segment (IS) and outer nuclear layer (ONL) of P10 *^{emb}Kif3a^{+/-}* photoreceptors, but was undetectable in *^{emb}Kif3a^{-/-}* photoreceptors (Fig. **4A**, right). At P10, newly synthesized rhodopsin actively trafficked toward the

$^{emb}Kif3a^{+/-}$ nascent ROS (Fig. **4B**, left), whereas rhodopsin continued to accumulate in the $^{emb}Kif3a^{-/-}$ ONL and IS (Fig. **4B**, right).

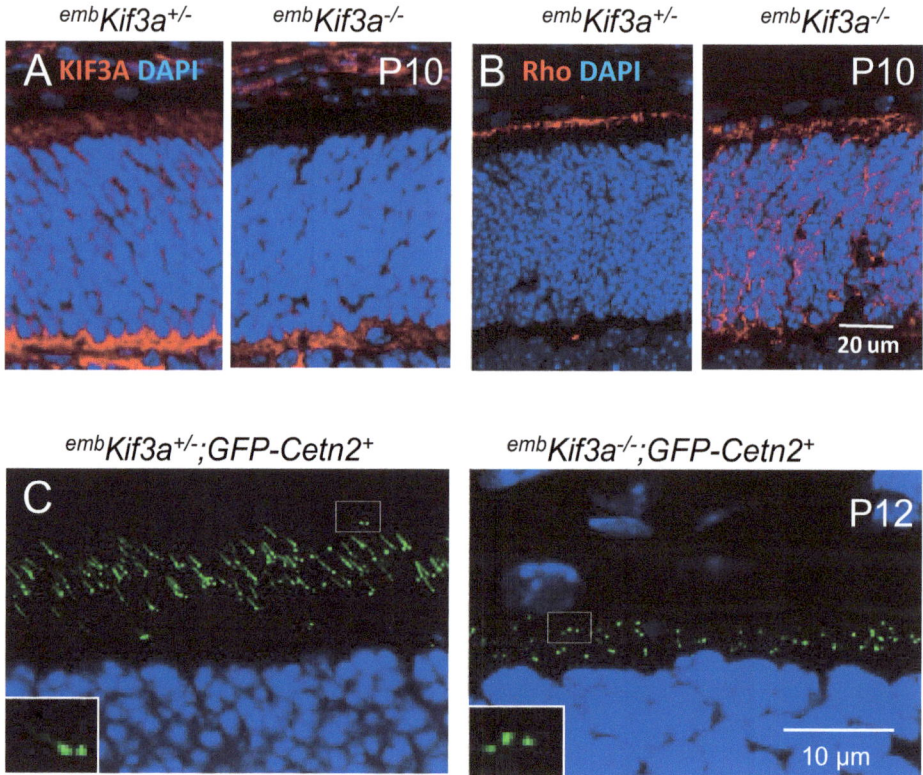

Fig. (4). Failure of OS formation in $^{emb}Kif3a^{-/-}$ rods. (A) KIF3A expression (red) in $^{emb}Kif3a^{+/-}$ (left) and $^{emb}Kif3a^{-/-}$ (right) photoreceptors. **(B)** Rhodopsin localization in $^{emb}Kif3a^{+/-}$ (left) and $^{emb}Kif3a^{-/-}$ (right) retinas. Rhodopsin mislocalizes to rod cell body of P10 $^{emb}Kif3a^{-/-}$ mice (right). **(C)** In $^{emb}Kif3a^{+/-}$; *EGFP-Cetn2*$^{+}$photoreceptors, centrioles appear as green dots and connecting cilia as 1μm-long green streaks. Only green "dot" centrioles are observed in $^{ret}Kif3a^{-/-}$ photoreceptors, indicating absence of CC and OS. In C, centrin-2 (CETN2) appears *via* transgene expression.

We investigated the formation of PTZs by fluorescence labeling with transgenic GFP-CETN2. CETN2 (centrin 2) is a Ca^{2+}-binding protein associated with photoreceptor centrioles and PTZs [17, 18]. Transgenic GFP-CETN2 fusion protein [19] expressed in $^{emb}Kif3a^{-/-}$; *Gfp-cetn2*$^{+}$ mice monitors the presence of basal bodies and PTZs (Fig. **2E**). By P12, fully developed PTZs are present (~1 μm in length), each paired with a daughter centriole at its base ("shooting star," Fig. (**4C**), left and inset). Apart from numerous centriolar pairs, no GFP-CENT2-labeled PTZs are detectable in $^{emb}Kif3a^{-/-}$ photoreceptor apical ISs (Fig. **4C**, right).

Tamoxifen-Induced KIF3A Depletion in the Adult Mouse

A rod-specific knockout of *Kif3a* showed that rhodopsin trafficked to the OSs even as they degenerated [14]. However, KIF3 was associated with rhodopsin trafficking in cultured hTert-RPE1 cells [20] and rhodopsin was pulled down by IFT88 together with GC1 as IFT cargo [21] suggesting involvement of KIF3 in rhodopsin trafficking. To solve this apparent discrepancy, we deleted KIF3A in the adult mouse using a tamoxifen-inducible *Cre/loxP* recombination system *CAG-CreET* [22]. We induced nuclear translocation of *CreET* with tamoxifen on five consecutive days and followed the rate of degeneration in cryosections for 8 weeks (Fig. **5A**). *Kif3a$^{f/-}$;CreET^{+}* (^{tam}*Kif3a$^{-/-}$*) photoreceptors degenerated progressively, but the rate of degeneration was slower and less severe than that occurring in ^{emb}*Kif3a$^{-/-}$* mice. At 2 weeks post-tamoxifen induction (PTI), no morphological defects were obvious in the ^{tam}*Kif3a$^{-/-}$* mouse retinas (Fig. **5A**, right). The OS shortened at 4 weeks PTI, and the degeneration progressed with reduction of photoreceptor OS lengths and ONL thickness (Fig. **5A**).

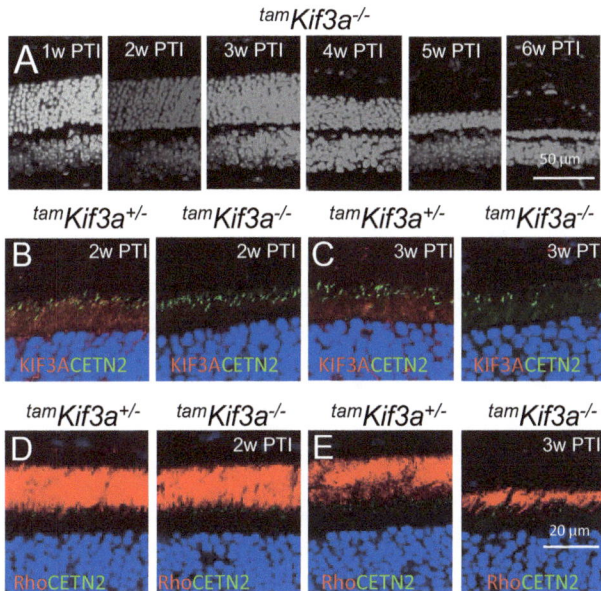

Fig. (5). Rhodopsin trafficking persists in KIF3A-depleted rods. (A) Retina transverse sections of *Kif3a* knockouts (^{tam}*Kif3a$^{-/-}$*) at 1w to 6wPTI. (**B, C**) KIF3A in ^{tam}*Kif3a$^{+/-}$* (left) and ^{tam}*Kif3a$^{-/-}$* (right) photoreceptors. KIF3A (red) is absent in ^{tam}*Kif3a$^{-/-}$* (right) photoreceptors at one to three weeks post-tamoxifen induction (1-3w PTI). (**D, E**) Rhodopsin in ^{tam}*Kif3a$^{+/-}$* (left) and ^{tam}*Kif3a$^{-/-}$*(right) rods. Rhodopsin (red) traffics normally even as the OS shorten and degenerate (D, right). Rhodopsin mislocalizes within the distal IS at 3w PTI. In B-E, centrin-2 (CETN2) was expressed transgenically.

Rhodopsin Traffics to ^{tam}*Kif3a$^{-/-}$* rod Outer Segments

If rhodopsin requires KIF3 to be transported from the inner to the OS, depletion of

KIF3A should cause rhodopsin mistrafficking. After five consecutive daily tamoxifen inductions of *Kif3a^f/-^;CreET^+^* mice, KIF3A was undetectable in the *^tam^Kif3a^-/-^* photoreceptors as early as one week PTI (not shown) counting from the first day of injection. In the *^tam^Kif3a^-/+^* controls, KIF3A levels were unchanged (Fig. **5B, 5C**, left). Rhodopsin localized normally in *^tam^Kif3a^-/-^* ROS at 1 and 2 weeks PTI (Fig. **5D**, right), a time interval during which ROS disc membranes should have been replaced completely. By three weeks PTI when the *^tam^Kif3a^-/-^* OS layer was shortened more than 50% (Fig. **5E**, right), rhodopsin was still localized correctly to the ROS although minor mislocalization of rhodopsin became obvious.

Homodimeric Kinesin-2 (KIF17) is not Essential for Photoreceptor IFT

Homodimeric KIF17 (Osm-3) is an alternate kinesin-2 motor that coordinates with KIF3 in anterograde IFT transport [10, 23]. To test whether KIF17 also participates in photoreceptor IFT, especially rhodopsin trafficking, we deleted exon 4 of the *Kif17* gene using a *Cre*/loxP gene targeting approach that truncates KIF17 protein after its motor domain (Fig. **6A**).

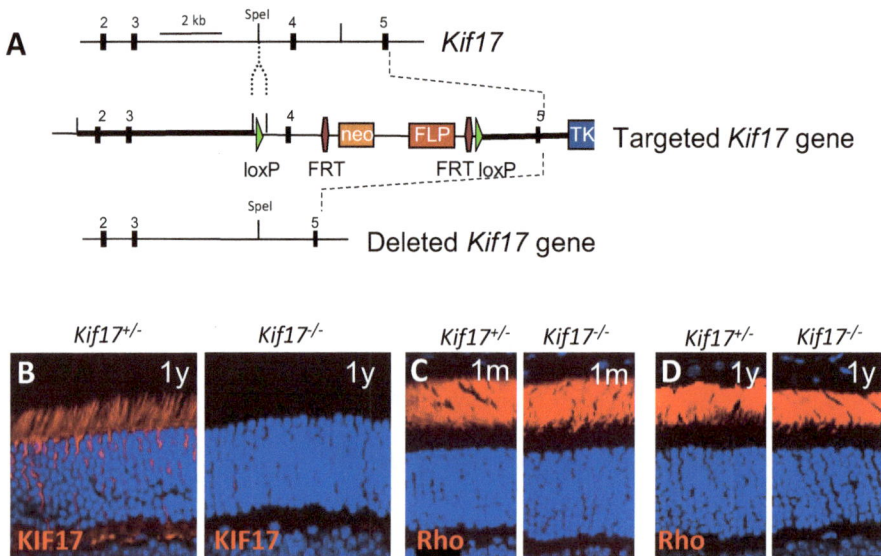

Fig. (6). Germline deletion of mouse *Kif17*. (A) Confirmation of KIF17 depletion in mouse photoreceptors by immunohistochemistry. In *Kif17^-/-^* retina, no KIF17 expression was observed. (B) Immunolocalization of rhodopsin. In Kif17^-/-^ mouse (right), rhodopsin targets to ROS at one month (top) and one year (bottom) of age.

Immunohistochemistry with anti-KIF17 antibodies verified absence of KIF17 in *Kif17^-/-^* mouse retina (Fig. **6B**). The knockout mice were healthy, fertile and indistinguishable from wild type mice. *Kif17^-/-^* retinal morphology was normal at all ages analyzed (1, 3, 6 and 12 months) not shown). Rhodopsin traffics to the OS in both one-month (Fig. **6B**, right) and one-year old *Kif17* knockout mice (Fig. **6C**, right).

To test whether KIF3 and KIF17 function redundantly in rhodopsin transport *via* IFT, we generated a rod-specific *Kif3a* and germline *Kif17* double knockout mouse, *iCre75⁺;Kif3a^{f/f};Kif17^{-/-}* (rod dKO), by crossing the ^{rod}*Kif3a^{-/-}* rod-specific knockout (*iCre75⁺;Kif3a^{f/f}*) [14] with the *Kif17^{-/-}* germline knockout mice. By immunohistochemistry, we observed normal rhodopsin transport to the OSs of P14 and P21 ^{rod}dKO mice (Fig. **7A, 7B**, right), as in the ^{rod}*Kif3a^{-/-};Kif17^{+/-}* controls. These results indicate that KIF17 and KIF3 do affect rhodopsin transport synergistically as neither single knockouts, nor KIF17/KIF3a double-knockout mice cause rhodopsin mistrafficking during rod senescence.

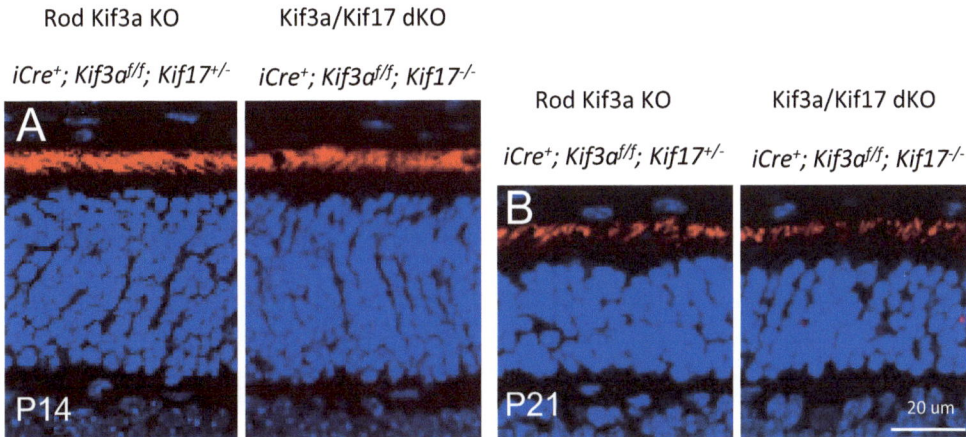

Fig. (7). Double Knockout of *Kif17* and *Kif3a* in Rods. Left panels, rhodopsin localization in*iCre75⁺; Kif3a^{f/f}; Kif17^{+/-}* (rod KIF3A knockout) retina. Right panel, rhodopsin localization in *iCre75⁺; Kif3a^{f/f}; Kif17^{-/-}* (Kif3a/*Kif17* double KO) retinas at P14 (**A**), and P21 (**B**).

CONCLUDING REMARKS

Our results show that deletion of KIF3A in retinal progenitors prevented connecting cilium/transition zone (CC/TZ), axoneme and OS formation in rod and cone photoreceptors, thus aborting ciliogenesis at a late stage. Deletion of KIF3A caused rapid photoreceptor degeneration starting at P10, and the degeneration was complete within 2 weeks (Fig. **2A**).

Extension of ciliary stalks and OS formation usually initiate around P3 and P7, respectively [24]. Expression of the basal body/PTZ marker GFP-CETN2 in ^{ret}*Kif3a^{-/-}* mice (Fig. **4C**) demonstrated absence of PTZs and axonemes. As a consequence of ciliogenesis arrest, newly synthesized rhodopsin destined to the

OSs backed up in the inner segments, photoreceptor axons and synaptic terminals (Fig. **4B**, right). These experiments show that IFT powered by KIF3 is required for PTZ formation and axoneme extension during retinal development.

In a second series of experiments, we depleted KIF3A and in fully developed photoreceptors of adult mice by tamoxifen-induced gene targeting (Figs. **5A** - **5E**). KIF3A was undetectable by immunohistochemistry in the ONL and inner segments one week after the first application of tamoxifen (not shown). Trafficking of rhodopsin proceeded normally in the absence of KIF3A for about three weeks after tamoxifen-induction (Fig. **5D, 5E**), even after onset of OS degeneration. This finding is consistent with our previous report [14] in which transgenic expression of Cre (iCre75) in rods caused OS degeneration, but did not interfere with rhodopsin trafficking. Apparently, membrane protein trafficking does not require KIF3 in rods. Renewal of both rod and cone OSs, accomplished every ten days and requiring re-synthesis of 80 OSs disks every day [25], proceeded normally in the absence of KIF3A.

Homodimeric kinesin-2 (KIF17) was reported to function as an anterograde IFT motor in mammalian cells transporting Sonic hedgehog signaling membrane proteins into cilia [26]. Knockdown of zebrafish *Kif17* disrupted targeting of visual pigment to the OSs [6], and KIF17 was also identified as a molecular motor transporting mouse olfactory channel subunits to cilia [27]. However, our germline *Kif17* knockout mouse had normal photoreceptor function at one month and one year of age, as documented by normal retina morphology at one year (**Fig. 6**). A $^{rod}KIF3a^{-/-};Kif17^{-/-}$ mouse, representing a rod *KIF3a/Kif17* double knockout (Fig. **7A, 7B**), replicated the rod degeneration phenotype observed with the $^{rod}KIF3a^{-/-}$ mouse, thereby excluding synergistic roles of homodimeric and heterotrimeric kinesin in rhodopsin trafficking.

In summary, *Kif3a* conditional knockout in mouse retina progenitors prevents rod/cone axoneme formation and OS morphogenesis. Tamoxifen-induced KIF3A deletion in the adult mouse impedes photoreceptor axoneme maintenance leading to progressive OS shortening from distal-to-proximal with subsequent photoreceptor degeneration. These experiments demonstrate collectively that kinesin-2 molecular motors are nonessential for ciliary trafficking of rhodopsin, cone pigments or other membrane-associated OS proteins. Consequently, IFT powered by heterotrimeric kinesin-2 is critical for axoneme maintenance.

MATERIALS AND METHODS

Mice. Mouse strains, genotyping and generation of mouse knockouts have been described [28, 29]. All experiments were approved by the Institutional Animal Care and Use Committee (IACUC) of the University of Utah, in compliance with statements for animal use of the Association for Research in Vision and Ophthalmology (ARVO). Mice were maintained under 12-hour cyclic dark/light conditions.

Antibodies. Rabbit anti-KIF3A (K3513; Sigma-Aldrich), rabbit anti-KIF17 (ab11261; Abcam), as well as antibodies directed against photoreceptor OS proteins and synaptic terminal proteins were described previously [14, 30].

Immunohistochemistry. Mouse eyecups were dissected and immediately immersion-fixed using 4% paraformaldeheyde in 0.1 M phosphate buffer, pH 7.4, for 2 hours on ice as described [31].

CONFLICT OF INTEREST

The author (editor) declares no conflict of interest, financial or otherwise.

ACKNOWLEDGEMENTS

This work was supported by NIH grants EY08123, EY019298 (WB), EY014800-039003 (NEI core grant), unrestricted grants to the Departments of Ophthalmology at the University of Utah from Research to Prevent Blindness (RPB; New York). WB is a recipient of a Research to Prevent Blindness Senior Investigator Award.

REFERENCES

[1]   Insinna C, Besharse JC. Intraflagellar transport and the sensory outer segment of vertebrate photoreceptors. Dev Dyn 2008; 237(8): 1982-92.
[http://dx.doi.org/10.1002/dvdy.21554] [PMID: 18489002]

[2]   Scholey JM. Cilium assembly: delivery of tubulin by kinesin-2-powered trains. Curr Biol 2013; 23(21): R956-9.
[http://dx.doi.org/10.1016/j.cub.2013.09.032] [PMID: 24200322]

[3]   Rosenbaum JL, Witman GB. Intraflagellar transport. Nat Rev Mol Cell Biol 2002; 3(11): 813-25.
[http://dx.doi.org/10.1038/nrm952] [PMID: 12415299]

[4]   Scholey JM. Kinesin-2: a family of heterotrimeric and homodimeric motors with diverse intracellular transport functions. Annu Rev Cell Dev Biol 2013; 29: 443-69.
[http://dx.doi.org/10.1146/annurev-cellbio-101512-122335] [PMID: 23750925]

[5]   Cole DG, Cande WZ, Baskin RJ, Skoufias DA, Hogan CJ, Scholey JM. Isolation of a sea urchin egg kinesin-related protein using peptide antibodies. J Cell Sci 1992; 101(Pt 2): 291-301.
[PMID: 1629246]

[6]   Insinna C, Pathak N, Perkins B, Drummond I, Besharse JC. The homodimeric kinesin, Kif17, is essential for vertebrate photoreceptor sensory outer segment development. Dev Biol 2008; 316(1): 160-70.
[http://dx.doi.org/10.1016/j.ydbio.2008.01.025] [PMID: 18304522]

[7]   Cole DG, Diener DR, Himelblau AL, Beech PL, Fuster JC, Rosenbaum JL. Chlamydomonas kinesin-II-dependent intraflagellar transport (IFT): IFT particles contain proteins required for ciliary assembly in Caenorhabditis elegans sensory neurons. J Cell Biol 1998; 141(4): 993-1008.

[http://dx.doi.org/10.1083/jcb.141.4.993] [PMID: 9585417]

[8]   Baker SA, Freeman K, Luby-Phelps K, Pazour GJ, Besharse JC. IFT20 links kinesin II with a mammalian intraflagellar transport complex that is conserved in motile flagella and sensory cilia. J Biol Chem 2003; 278(36): 34211-8.
[http://dx.doi.org/10.1074/jbc.M300156200] [PMID: 12821668]

[9]   Muresan V, Lyass A, Schnapp BJ. The kinesin motor KIF3A is a component of the presynaptic ribbon in vertebrate photoreceptors. J Neurosci 1999; 19(3): 1027-37.
[PMID: 9920666]

[10]   Signor D, Wedaman KP, Rose LS, Scholey JM. Two heteromeric kinesin complexes in chemosensory neurons and sensory cilia of Caenorhabditis elegans. Mol Biol Cell 1999; 10(2): 345-60.
[http://dx.doi.org/10.1091/mbc.10.2.345] [PMID: 9950681]

[11]   Pan X, Ou G, Civelekoglu-Scholey G, *et al.* Mechanism of transport of IFT particles in C. elegans cilia by the concerted action of kinesin-II and OSM-3 motors. J Cell Biol 2006; 174(7): 1035-45.
[http://dx.doi.org/10.1083/jcb.200606003] [PMID: 17000880]

[12]   Marszalek JR, Liu X, Roberts EA, *et al.* Genetic evidence for selective transport of opsin and arrestin by kinesin-II in mammalian photoreceptors. Cell 2000; 102(2): 175-87.
[http://dx.doi.org/10.1016/S0092-8674(00)00023-4] [PMID: 10943838]

[13]   Jimeno D, Feiner L, Lillo C, *et al.* Analysis of kinesin-2 function in photoreceptor cells using synchronous Cre-loxP knockout of Kif3a with RHO-Cre. Invest Ophthalmol Vis Sci 2006; 47(11): 5039-46.
[http://dx.doi.org/10.1167/iovs.06-0032] [PMID: 17065525]

[14]   Avasthi P, Watt CB, Williams DS, *et al.* Trafficking of membrane proteins to cone but not rod outer segments is dependent on heterotrimeric kinesin-II. J Neurosci 2009; 29(45): 14287-98.
[http://dx.doi.org/10.1523/JNEUROSCI.3976-09.2009] [PMID: 19906976]

[15]   Malicki J, Besharse JC. Kinesin-2 family motors in the unusual photoreceptor cilium. Vision Res 2012; 75: 33-6.
[http://dx.doi.org/10.1016/j.visres.2012.10.008] [PMID: 23123805]

[16]   Furuta Y, Lagutin O, Hogan BL, Oliver GC. Retina- and ventral forebrain-specific Cre recombinase activity in transgenic mice. Genesis 2000; 26(2): 130-2.
[http://dx.doi.org/10.1002/(SICI)1526-968X(200002)26:2<130::AID-GENE9>3.0.CO;2-I] [PMID: 10686607]

[17]   Giessl A, Trojan P, Rausch S, Pulvermüller A, Wolfrum U. Centrins, gatekeepers for the light-dependent translocation of transducin through the photoreceptor cell connecting cilium. Vision Res 2006; 46(27): 4502-9.
[http://dx.doi.org/10.1016/j.visres.2006.07.029] [PMID: 17027897]

[18]   Ying G, Avasthi P, Irwin M, *et al.* Centrin 2 is required for mouse olfactory ciliary trafficking and development of ependymal cilia planar polarity. J Neurosci 2014; 34(18): 6377-88.
[http://dx.doi.org/10.1523/JNEUROSCI.0067-14.2014] [PMID: 24790208]

[19]   Higginbotham H, Bielas S, Tanaka T, Gleeson JG. Transgenic mouse line with green-fluorescent protein-labeled Centrin 2 allows visualization of the centrosome in living cells. Transgenic Res 2004; 13(2): 155-64.
[http://dx.doi.org/10.1023/B:TRAG.0000026071.41735.8e] [PMID: 15198203]

[20]   Trivedi D, Colin E, Louie CM, Williams DS. Live-cell imaging evidence for the ciliary transport of rod photoreceptor opsin by heterotrimeric kinesin-2. J Neurosci 2012; 32(31): 10587-93.
[http://dx.doi.org/10.1523/JNEUROSCI.0015-12.2012] [PMID: 22855808]

[21]   Bhowmick R, Li M, Sun J, Baker SA, Insinna C, Besharse JC. Photoreceptor IFT complexes containing chaperones, guanylyl cyclase 1 and rhodopsin. Traffic 2009; 10(6): 648-63.
[http://dx.doi.org/10.1111/j.1600-0854.2009.00896.x] [PMID: 19302411]

[22]   Hayashi S, McMahon AP. Efficient recombination in diverse tissues by a tamoxifen-inducible form of Cre: a tool for temporally regulated gene activation/inactivation in the mouse. Dev Biol 2002; 244(2): 305-18.
[http://dx.doi.org/10.1006/dbio.2002.0597] [PMID: 11944939]

[23]   Scholey JM. Kinesin-2 motors transport IFT-particles, dyneins and tubulin subunits to the tips of Caenorhabditis elegans sensory cilia: relevance to vision research? Vision Res 2012; 75: 44-52.
[http://dx.doi.org/10.1016/j.visres.2012.06.015] [PMID: 22772029]

[24]   Olney JW. An electron microscopic study of synapse formation, receptor outer segment development, and other aspects of developing mouse retina. Invest Ophthalmol 1968; 7(3): 250-68.
[PMID: 5655873]

[25]   Young RW. Visual cells and the concept of renewal. Invest Ophthalmol Vis Sci 1976; 15(9): 700-25.
[PMID: 986765]

[26]   Liem KF Jr, He M, Ocbina PJ, Anderson KV. Mouse Kif7/Costal2 is a cilia-associated protein that regulates Sonic hedgehog signaling. Proc Natl Acad Sci USA 2009; 106(32): 13377-82.
[http://dx.doi.org/10.1073/pnas.0906944106] [PMID: 19666503]

[27]   Jenkins PM, Hurd TW, Zhang L, *et al.* Ciliary targeting of olfactory CNG channels requires the CNGB1b subunit and the kinesin-2 motor protein, KIF17. Curr Biol 2006; 16(12): 1211-6.
[http://dx.doi.org/10.1016/j.cub.2006.04.034] [PMID: 16782012]

[28]   Jiang L, Wei Y, Ronquillo CC, *et al.* Heterotrimeric kinesin-2 (KIF3) mediates transition zone and axoneme formation of mouse photoreceptors. J Biol Chem 2015; 290(20): 12765-78.
[http://dx.doi.org/10.1074/jbc.M115.638437] [PMID: 25825494]

[29]   Jiang L, Tam BM, Ying G, Wu S, Hauswirth WW, Frederick JM, *et al.* KIF17 (Osm-3): a Vestigial Anterograde Kinesin-2 Motor. J Biol Chem 2015. under revision

[30]   Baehr W, Karan S, Maeda T, *et al.* The function of guanylate cyclase 1 and guanylate cyclase 2 in rod and cone photoreceptors. J Biol Chem 2007; 282(12): 8837-47.
[http://dx.doi.org/10.1074/jbc.M610369200] [PMID: 17255100]

[31]   Jiang L, Zhang H, Dizhoor AM, *et al.* Long-term RNA interference gene therapy in a dominant retinitis pigmentosa mouse model. Proc Natl Acad Sci USA 2011; 108(45): 18476-81.
[http://dx.doi.org/10.1073/pnas.1112758108] [PMID: 22042849]

CHAPTER 6

The Molecular Links between Mutations in RDS and Diseases of the Retina

Michael W. Stuck, Shannon M. Conley and **Muna I. Naash**[*]

Department of Cell Biology, University of Oklahoma Health Sciences Center, Oklahoma City, Oklahoma, USA

Abstract: The photoreceptor specific tetraspanin protein peripherin-2, also known as retinal degeneration slow (RDS) plays a critical role in the biogenesis and maintenance of both rod and cone photoreceptor outer segments. Over 80 pathological mutations in RDS have been linked with multiple degenerative blinding diseases including retinitis pigmentosa and various forms of macular degeneration. RDS-associated disease is characterized by a diverse set of phenotypes with variability in penetrance, severity, and timing of disease onset. Much insight into the complex pathological mechanisms associated with RDS mutations has been gleaned from work in animal models with disease-causing mutations. In the current review we summarize our current understanding of RDS function in the normal retina and how defects in this function contribute to the associated disease pathologies in human patients.

Keywords: Animal models, Blindness, Choriocapillaris atrophy, Cones, Disease mechanisms, Electroretinography, Macular dystrophy, Microdomain, Morphogenesis, Outer segments, Photoreceptors, Protein complexes, Protein trafficking, RDS, Retinal degeneration, Retinitis pigmentosa, Rim region, Rods, ROM-1, Tetraspanin.

INTRODUCTION

Peripherin-2, also known as retinal degeneration slow (RDS), is a photoreceptor-specific tetraspanin and is necessary for the formation of rod and cone outer segments (OSs) [1 - 7]. More than 80 pathogenic mutations in the human RDS gene (PRPH2) have been identified and lead to a diverse set of mostly dominantly inherited retinal degenerative diseases [8]. RDS-associated pathologies can be broadly characterized as either retinitis pigmentosa (RP), which primarily affects rod photoreceptor cells, or macular dystrophies (MD), which primarily affect central vision, either by direct effects on cone photoreceptors or by causing signi-

[*] **Corresponding author Muna I. Naash:** Department of Biomedical Engineering, University of Houston, 3517 Cullen Blvd. Room 2027, Houston, TX 77204-5060, USA; Tel: 713-743-1651; E-mail: mnaash@central.uh.edu

Hemant Khanna (Ed)

ficant defects in neighboring tissues such as the retinal pigment epithelium (RPE)/choroid which result in macular vision loss [8 - 10]. An excellent resource for RDS-associated pathologies can be found on the Retina International website (http://www.retina-international.org/ files/sci-news/ /rdsmut.htm). Autosomal dominant RP (adRP) represents 20-40% of total cases of RP [11, 12]. Though rhodopsin mutations account for more adRP than any other gene (~25%) [11], RDS is one of the most common associated genes other than rhodopsin (~2.5-9% of adRP cases) [11, 12]. The pathology of MD is complex and represents a broad spectrum of disorders including pattern dystrophies, adult-onset foveomacular vitelliform dystrophy, central areolar choroidal dystrophy, AMD-like late onset MD and multifocal pattern dystrophy simulating STGD1/fundus flaviomaculatus [8], many of which have significant overlap in their clinical presentation. The percentage of MDs linked to RDS mutations ranges from 2-18% [8] depending on the population. A thorough understanding of the RDS protein and its molecular function in OS biogenesis is critical for developing treatments for these important blinding diseases. Here we focus on what is known of the molecular role of RDS in OS biogenesis and how interruption of these processes leads to disease pathology.

RDS PROTEIN, TERTIARY STRUCTURE AND COMPLEX FORMATION

Photoreceptor OSs are highly modified 9+0 primary cilia. The OSs contain hundreds of flattened membrane structures, termed discs in rods and lamellae in cones, which are organized and stacked mostly perpendicular to the incoming light [13]. The discs are encased in a sheath of the plasma membrane in rods but are at least partially contiguous with the plasma membranes in cones [14, 15]. Each flattened disc/lamellae is circumscribed by a rim region with a distinct hairpin structure [13, 14, 16]. RDS localizes to this rim region and plays a critical role in maintaining the curvature and general organization of this highly-ordered lipid structure [17 - 20].

The RDS protein is a 39 kD four pass transmembrane glycoprotein with cytosolic N- and C- termini and two asymmetrical loops (D1 and D2) which project into the intradiscal space in rods and the analogous lamellar lumen/extracellular space in cones [7, 21, 22]. The N-terminus, transmembrane domains and D1 loop of RDS are thought to function as the structural backbone allowing the proper folding and packing of RDS within the disc membrane [23] while the D2 loop and C-terminal domains have established functional roles. The D2 loop mediates covalent and non-covalent intermolecular interactions, facilitating oligomerization, and is the site of the sole RDS N-linked glycosylation [23]. The C-terminal of RDS is a multi-functional domain that helps target RDS to the OS, forms a binding domain for the GARP subunit of the rod (but not cone) cyclic nucleotide gated channel and melanoregulin, and forms an amphipathic helix involved in the regulation or generation of lipid curvature and membrane fusion in the OS [19, 20, 24 - 32].

Following synthesis, the RDS monomer associates with itself and with its homologue rod outer segment membrane protein 1 (ROM-1) to form both homo- and hetero-tetramers which are the core of the functional oligomers of RDS [33 - 35] (Fig. **1A**). ROM-1 shares a similar tertiary structure with RDS although it lacks any known functional domains within its C-terminus and is not glycosylated [36]. RDS is more abundant in OSs than ROM-1, and ROM-1 is thought to act primarily as an ancillary protein perhaps modulating RDS' function [23, 25, 37 - 39]. ROM-1 is capable of forming tetramers that do not include RDS, and pools of ROM-1 alone have been isolated in detergent resistant rafts from OSs, although no ROM-1 function independent of RDS has been identified [40, 41]. While RDS/RDS RDS/ROM-1 and ROM-1/ROM-1 tetramers are held together through non-covalent interactions, both RDS and ROM-1 also form intermolecular disulfide bonds mediated by a cysteine at position 150 and 153, respectively, within their D2 loops [42]. These intermolecular disulfide bonds allow RDS/RDS and RDS/ROM-1 tetramers to link up into larger oligomers, which are thought to form after exit from the ER, though oligomerization may occur differently in rods and cones [43, 44]. Both RDS and ROM-1 are found in non-covalent tetramers and in disulfide linked intermediate-sized complexes but the largest type of complexes contains only RDS [35, 42] (Fig. **1A**).

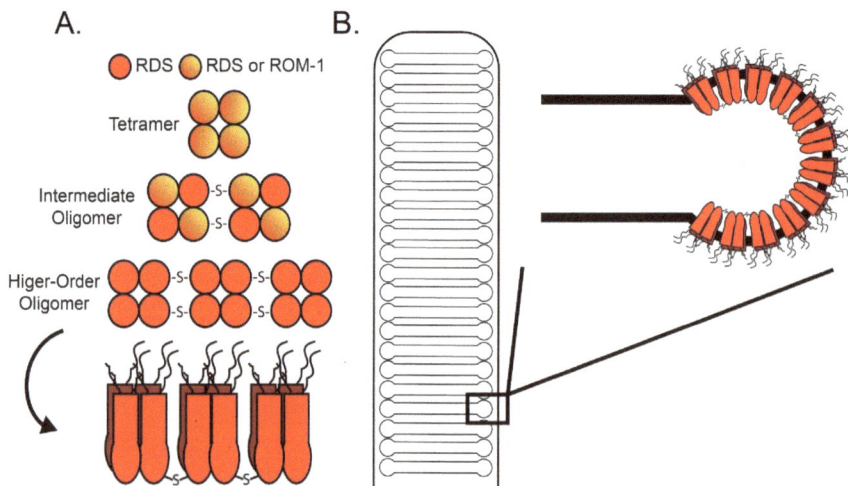

Fig. (1). Diagram describing RDS complex formation. A. RDS and ROM-1 assemble into covalent and non-covalent complexes. Red balls represent RDS and orange balls are either RDS or ROM-1. **B.** Model for assembly of RDS complexes in the membrane. RDS ability to mediate membrane curvature coupled with space measurements suggests that the complexes are oriented around the hairpin. **B** is modified from [20].

Covalently-linked RDS higher-order and intermediate complexes are necessary for RDS' function, as mutants incapable of forming intermolecular disulfide bonds do not form OSs [44 - 46]. In spite of the existence of these multiple different types of oligomers, clear roles for each complex type have not been identified. It was originally suggested that RDS disulfide bonding occurred across the lumen of the OS disc, however size and packing models for RDS/ROM-1 tetramers coupled with advanced measurements of OS/disc dimensions strongly support a model by which RDS/ROM-1 disulfide bond formation occurs laterally between neighboring tetramers of RDS/ROM-1 [20, 35], thus promoting membrane curvature (Fig. **1B**). In summary, through the formation of various types of oligomers, RDS/ROM-1 are thought to play a role in biogenesis of the OS through the promotion of membrane curvature and organization of the OS rims/rim microdomain.

RDS AND RETINITIS PIGMENTOSA

RP is a degenerative disease characterized by the initial loss of rod photoreceptors [8, 12]. This usually manifests as night blindness and the loss of peripheral to mid-peripheral vision [8, 12]. The loss of vision progresses at variable rates and eventually leads to loss of central vision and total blindness later in life [11]. RP-causing mutations in RDS are nearly universally inherited in an autosomal dominant fashion although digenic forms of the disease exist [47]. The majority of RDS-associated RP presents in the 3rd to 5th decades of life with loss of visual acuity occurring around 50 years of age, though there is a wide range in onset and severity of vision loss. As a rule, age of onset and overall severity of the disease are correlated [8]. Full-field electroretinography (ERG) usually shows an absence of rod response with a decrease in cone response ranging from mild to severe [8]. While most mutations lead to disease states in later life notable exceptions exist and include N244K, D173V, and P216L [8, 10]. In these cases, disease onset and vision loss are severe and can occur within the first decade of life.

RDS mutations lead to RP through loss-of-function and haploinsufficiency [38]. Our understanding of RDS haploinsufficiency has been aided by the *retinal degeneration slow* (*rds*) mouse (also known as *rds*$^{-/-}$ or *rd2*), which contains a naturally occurring *rds* null allele [1, 2, 6, 48]. In heterozygous mice (*rds*$^{+/-}$), the retina has close to the normal number of photoreceptors at one month of age, but exhibits slow degeneration over time with rods dying before cones, both through apoptosis [49]. Rod ERGs are significantly and progressively reduced throughout life while cone ERG responses are initially normal, or nearly so, followed by a gradual loss of signal [49]. This functional outcome has structural analogs. The *rds*$^{+/-}$ rod OSs fail to form properly and instead form abnormal whorl structures [5] (Fig. **2A**). Interestingly, this structure-function correlation is not preserved in cones. Immunogold labeling with short-wavelength cone opsin antibodies to identify cones shows that cone OS structure is also abnormal in the $rds^{+/-}$ from one month of age Fig. (**2B**) though defects in cone function are not observed until later, 4-6 months of age [49], suggesting that cones better tolerate alterations in OS structure than rods. Mouse models carrying RP mutations such as C214S suggest that the mutant protein is not stable and is degraded, consistent with a loss-of-function allele [50]. Taken together the phenotype observed in $rds^{+/-}$ mice almost exactly mimics the standard human pathology associated with the majority of RDS RP associated mutations.

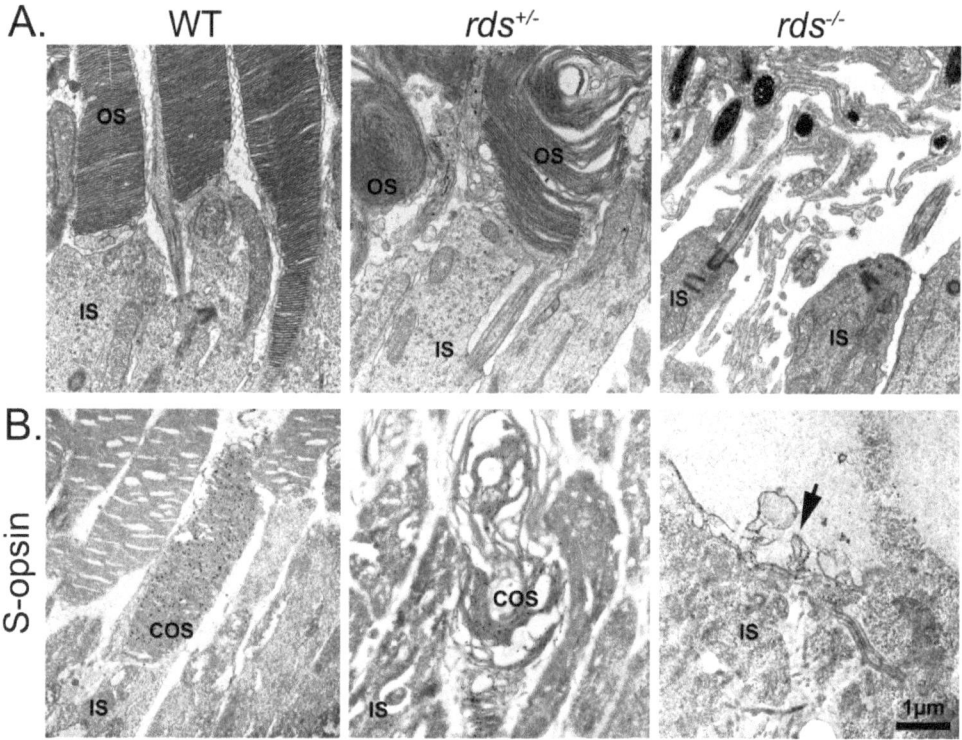

Fig. (2). **RDS haploinsufficiency leads to defects in rod and cone OS structure. A.** Shown are electron micrographs from the indicated genotypes at postnatal day 30 demonstrating abnormal OS formation in the $rds^{+/-}$ and no OS formation in the $rds^{-/-}$. **B.** Sections were immunolabeled with S-opsin antibodies to identify cone OSs. Observe abnormalities in cone OS formation in $rds^{+/-}$ retinas. Arrow indicates S-opsin labeled membranous material in the subretinal space in $rds^{-/-}$ but no OS formation. OS: outer segment, IS: inner segment, COS: cone outer segment. Scale bar: 1 μm.

The RDS null mouse ($rds^{-/-}$) has an even more severe phenotype. No OSs are formed at all and rod ERGs are undetectable [4] and cone ERG signal is extremely low. The $rds^{-/-}$ can serve as a model for some of the more severe forms of RP associated with RDS, because some RDS RP mutations lead to not only degradation of the mutant protein, but the remaining wild-type (WT) RDS as well. For example, a mouse model was generated in which the P216L RP mutation was expressed as a transgene on the $rds^{+/-}$ background [38]. This model carried a WT amount of RDS transcript (roughly 50% mutant and 50% WT), yet the total amount of RDS protein was reduced to only 8% of WT [38] with predictably severe structural and functional consequences [51]. Thus the total amount of RDS is further reduced than what would be predicted with a simple loss-of-function allele and is closer to the $rds^{-/-}$ than the $rds^{+/-}$. Consistent with this, patients with P216L mutations have more severe phenotypes than those with mutations associated with a single loss-of-function allele. The loss of RDS has a dose-dependent effect on photoreceptors with estimates suggesting that ~60-80% of WT levels of RDS are needed for normal rod OS biogenesis [38, 52]. When RDS levels drop below the threshold needed for OS biogenesis RP begins to manifest with increasing severity and earlier onset with greater degrees of RDS protein loss.

The link between RDS haploinsufficiency and the death of the rod photoreceptors through apoptosis remains poorly understood. Cone photoreceptors are also structurally and functionally defective in the absence of RDS, although to a lesser degree than rod photoreceptors; yet they are not subject to the same cell loss as rod cells [53, 54], thus the rod-then-cone nature of the RP diagnosis. Cone OS structure is different from rods, but at this time there is no clear model for why this would provide a survival advantage for the cone photoreceptors. It is worth noting that other RP associated mutations such as those in rhodopsin also eventually lead to the loss of cone photoreceptors despite having no primary impact on cones, consistent with survival interdependence between the two cell types.

RDS AND MACULAR DEGENERATION

In humans, high acuity central vision is mediated by the macula which contains the highest density of cone photoreceptors in the retina [15]. As the region responsible for most daytime vision, the macula experiences unique stresses that the peripheral retina is largely able to avoid [15, 55]. RDS-associated MD covers a broad spectrum of autosomal dominant diseases, first noticed as subtle defects in central vision starting in the 5th decade of life but can advance to very significant visual loss later in life [8]. There is a significant degree of inter and intra-familial phenotypic variability, both between mutations and between populations with the same mutation [56 - 58]. MD patients often exhibit various hypo or hyper-pigmented regions, which can be focal or multifocal in nature, and appear as yellow, orange or grey spots visible by funduscopic examination. These can remain as discrete lesions or grow over time and can have significant impacts on central vision [8]. Some mutations in RDS, such as R172W, are also associated with pigmentation defects of the RPE cells that over time lead to atrophy of the RPE and choriocapillaris and severe vision loss [10, 59, 60]. Patients are diagnosed with the varying forms of MD (pattern dystrophy, adult onset foveomacular vitelliform dystrophy, *etc.*) based upon timing of onset, the localization and nature of the observed pigmentation defects, and whether the disease is associated with atrophy of the RPE and choriocapillaris as well as choroidal neovascularization. The pathology of individual MD associated RDS mutations is likely influenced by the environment as well as secondary genetic traits, including polymorphisms in either ABCA4 or ROM-1 [61], though this may be specific to certain populations and certain RDS mutations [62].

In contrast to RP, all RDS MD mutations that have been examined thus far result in a protein capable of trafficking to the OS and forming at least some RDS oligomers [56, 63, 64]. The autosomal dominant inheritance of these disease mutations combined with stable protein products would suggest that these mutant proteins are acting primarily through a gain-of-function mechanism. This is supported by evidence from transgenic mice carrying MD mutations. For example, in the R172W transgenic model of MD cone function was significantly decreased while rod function was not, even in the presence of a full complement of WT RDS (*i.e.* transgenic on the WT background [65]). This phenomenon is not due to overexpression, as excess WT RDS is not damaging to photoreceptors [52]. As yet no region of RDS has been identified which convincingly imparts a cell specific (*i.e.* cone *versus* rod) function. In addition, different mutations in an amino acid (*e.g.* N244) can lead to either RP or MD: N224K results in adRP and rod-cone degeneration [66] while N224H is associated with MD/cone-rod dystrophy [67]. Work comparing RDS mutations expressed in tissue culture *versus* the same mutations expressed in photoreceptor cells suggest photoreceptors may have cell type specific chaperones, binding partners, or OS structures which allow for rod or cone specific effects [68], but these factors are not known.

One of the gain-of-function mechanisms for MD mutants is the generation of abnormal oligomers of RDS and ROM-1. For example, the cone specific MD mutation R172W induces the formation of abnormal intermediate-sized complexes containing ROM-1 preferentially in cones [63]. Though it is not clear why the biochemistry of R172W should be different in cones vs. rods, there is precedence for differences in the role of RDS oligomers in the two cell types [44, 46]. Funduscopic examination revealed that in addition to the cone-dominant ERG defect, R172W transgenic mice recapitulated some of the complicated phenotypes occurring in human patients with the R172W mutation including retinal degeneration, RPE defects, and defects in the choroid and vasculature [63]. In comparison, a knock-in mouse model carrying the Y141C MD mutation in the native RDS allele resulted in a distinctly different phenotype and defect in complex formation [56]. In this model both WT and mutant RDS as well as ROM-1 were found in very large complexes that exceed the usual size of the largest RDS complexes in both rods and cones [56]. The presence of ROM-1 in these complexes is of special note since ROM-1 is not normally found in large RDS homooligomers [35, 43]. These complexes are visible only under non-reducing conditions suggesting that the Y141C mutation leads to the formation of additional intermolecular disulfide bridges that contribute to the formation of abnormal RDS complexes [56]. In contrast to the R172W, the Y141C did not display the same tendency for RPE and choroid defects, but instead was characterized by the appearance of multi-focal hyper-fluorescent yellow flecks that were spread throughout the entire retina [56]. In both cases primary defects were observed in the photoreceptor cells themselves while secondary effects were observed in the neighboring RPE cells; both hallmarks of the MD pathology observed in patients.

Abnormal RDS oligomerization provides an attractive model to explain part of the phenotypic variability between individual MD associated mutations. Subtle differences in the tertiary structure of RDS caused by individual MD-associated mutations could have drastic effects on the formation, stability, or shape of higher order RDS oligomers, thus disrupting membrane curvature (as in Fig. **1B**). While it is not clear why RDS oligomerization defects would have a more significant impact on cone photoreceptors than rods, it is worth noting that the discs in rod photoreceptors are isolated from the plasma membranes while the lamellae of the cones are more dynamic and are thought to be contiguous with the plasma membrane and possibly undergo membrane fusion/fission events [15]. It is possible that the isolations of oligomers within the discs themselves helps protect the rods from oligomerization defects while the dynamic nature of cone OSs contributes to their sensitivity to RDS oligomer defects although without clear experimental testing this remains mostly conjecture.

The presence of abnormal RDS complexes in photoreceptor OSs might also help explain the observed secondary effects on the RPE if they are not properly degraded after OS phagocytosis. The ability of the RPE and photoreceptors to handle these complexes would be heavily dependent on potential secondary genetic traits that modulate cellular processes such as phagocytosis, lysosomal breakdown of OS constituents, export of protein aggregates and immune responses. Subtle changes in all of these processes could contribute to the variability in disease progression and severity in patients with RDS mutations. With additional testing the pathways and processes which contribute to the development of RDS associated MD patients should become clearer.

CONCLUDING REMARKS

Regardless of the exact nature and molecular mechanisms of RDS-associated disease our primary goal is to understand how to cure these diseases in human patients. The fact that RP is primarily associated with a loss of the RDS protein makes it a target for gene replacement therapy and many proof-of-principle experiments have shown the viability of this approach [69 - 72]. The primary obstacles remain efficient transfection of the photoreceptors and sustained expression of RDS-expressing constructs. While gene therapy would correct the primary defect, alternative approaches could include simply limiting the rate of cell loss in these diseases. Work in mice has shown that even in the complete absence of RDS and OS structure some vision remains as long as the photoreceptor itself is not lost [73]. It is possible that significant improvement in overall quality of life could be gained for patients by simply preventing cell loss by blocking apoptosis or providing other factors that help preserve the retina itself, and neurotrophic therapies have been evaluated with mixed results [74 - 77]. On the other hand, RDS-associated MD has a more complex disease mechanism and as such likely will require more complex interventions. While gene supplementation with WT RDS has shown benefit, it was transient and incomplete [68], and the gain-of-function nature of the associated mutations would imply that the mutant allele either needs to be eliminated or the gain-o--function defects need to be blocked through some other means. It is likely that a combination of gene supplementation with WT RDS along with pharmacological interventions to protect the health of the RPE and prevent cell loss will combine to help slow or prevent disease progression in patients.

A significant amount of work remains to be done. RDS mutations associated with MD especially require further study to determine how changes to RDS oligomers lead to the downstream phenotypes observed and to determine if factors other than complex formation contribute to the gain-of-function nature of these mutations. It is worth noting that all of the observed abnormal complexes seen in MD models so far have involved drastic changes to ROM-1. This highlights the importance of work to further characterize the role of ROM-1. The cellular pathways that lead to cell death for both RP and MD in photoreceptors and RPE cells remain especially poorly understood and characterized. The importance of RDS to photoreceptor structure and the prevalence of RDS mutations in human visual diseases make further work on the RDS molecule an important avenue of vision research for the foreseeable future.

ABBREVIATIONS

ADRP   Autosomal Dominant Retinitis Pigmentosa

ERG   Electroretinography

MD   Macular Dystrophies

OS   Outer Segments

RDS   Retinal Degeneration Slow

ROM-1 Rod Outer Segment Membrane Protein-1

RP   Retinitis Pigmentosa

RPE   Retinal Pigment Epithelium

WT   Wild-type.

CONFLICT OF INTEREST

The author (editor) declares no conflict of interest, financial or otherwise.

ACKNOWLEDGEMENTS

This work was supported by the National Institutes of Health (EY010609, EY22778, EY018656-MIN, T32EY023202-MWS), the Foundation Fighting Blindness (MIN), and the Oklahoma Center for the Advancement of Science and Technology (SMC). The S-opsin antibody was generously shared by Dr. Cheryl Craft, University of Southern California.

REFERENCES

[1]   van Nie R, Iványi D, Démant P. A new H-2-linked mutation, rds, causing retinal degeneration in the mouse. Tissue Antigens 1978; 12(2): 106-8.
[http://dx.doi.org/10.1111/j.1399-0039.1978.tb01305.x] [PMID: 705766]

[2]   Démant P, Iványi D, van Nie R. The map position of the rds gene on the 17th chromosome of the mouse. Tissue Antigens 1979; 13(1): 53-5.
[http://dx.doi.org/10.1111/j.1399-0039.1979.tb01136.x] [PMID: 419532]

[3]   Sanyal S, Jansen HG. Absence of receptor outer segments in the retina of rds mutant mice. Neurosci Lett 1981; 21(1): 23-6.
[http://dx.doi.org/10.1016/0304-3940(81)90051-3] [PMID: 7207866]

[4]   Reuter JH, Sanyal S. Development and degeneration of retina in rds mutant mice: the electroretinogram. Neurosci Lett 1984; 48(2): 231-7.
[http://dx.doi.org/10.1016/0304-3940(84)90024-7] [PMID: 6483282]

[5]   Hawkins RK, Jansen HG, Sanyal S. Development and degeneration of retina in rds mutant mice: photoreceptor abnormalities in the heterozygotes. Exp Eye Res 1985; 41(6): 701-20.
[http://dx.doi.org/10.1016/0014-4835(85)90179-4] [PMID: 3830736]

[6]   Travis GH, Brennan MB, Danielson PE, Kozak CA, Sutcliffe JG. Identification of a photoreceptor-specific mRNA encoded by the gene responsible for retinal degeneration slow (rds). Nature 1989; 338(6210): 70-3.
[http://dx.doi.org/10.1038/338070a0] [PMID: 2918924]

[7]   Connell G, Bascom R, Molday L, Reid D, McInnes RR, Molday RS. Photoreceptor peripherin is the

normal product of the gene responsible for retinal degeneration in the rds mouse. Proc Natl Acad Sci USA 1991; 88(3): 723-6.
[http://dx.doi.org/10.1073/pnas.88.3.723] [PMID: 1992463]

[8]   Boon CJ, den Hollander AI, Hoyng CB, Cremers FP, Klevering BJ, Keunen JE. The spectrum of retinal dystrophies caused by mutations in the peripherin/RDS gene. Prog Retin Eye Res 2008; 27(2): 213-35.
[http://dx.doi.org/10.1016/j.preteyeres.2008.01.002] [PMID: 18328765]

[9]   Kajiwara K, Hahn LB, Mukai S, Travis GH, Berson EL, Dryja TP. Mutations in the human retinal degeneration slow gene in autosomal dominant retinitis pigmentosa. Nature 1991; 354(6353): 480-3.
[http://dx.doi.org/10.1038/354480a0] [PMID: 1684223]

[10]   Wells J, Wroblewski J, Keen J, *et al.* Mutations in the human retinal degeneration slow (RDS) gene can cause either retinitis pigmentosa or macular dystrophy. Nat Genet 1993; 3(3): 213-8.
[http://dx.doi.org/10.1038/ng0393-213] [PMID: 8485576]

[11]   Hartong DT, Berson EL, Dryja TP. Retinitis pigmentosa. Lancet 2006; 368(9549): 1795-809.
[http://dx.doi.org/10.1016/S0140-6736(06)69740-7] [PMID: 17113430]

[12]   Ferrari S, Di Iorio E, Barbaro V, Ponzin D, Sorrentino FS, Parmeggiani F. Retinitis pigmentosa: genes and disease mechanisms. Curr Genomics 2011; 12(4): 238-49.
[http://dx.doi.org/10.2174/138920211795860107] [PMID: 22131869]

[13]   Sung CH, Chuang JZ. The cell biology of vision. J Cell Biol 2010; 190(6): 953-63.
[http://dx.doi.org/10.1083/jcb.201006020] [PMID: 20855501]

[14]   Carter-Dawson LD, LaVail MM. Rods and cones in the mouse retina. I. Structural analysis using light and electron microscopy. J Comp Neurol 1979; 188(2): 245-62.
[http://dx.doi.org/10.1002/cne.901880204] [PMID: 500858]

[15]   Mustafi D, Engel AH, Palczewski K. Structure of cone photoreceptors. Prog Retin Eye Res 2009; 28(4): 289-302.
[http://dx.doi.org/10.1016/j.preteyeres.2009.05.003] [PMID: 19501669]

[16]   Steinberg RH, Fisher SK, Anderson DH. Disc morphogenesis in vertebrate photoreceptors. J Comp Neurol 1980; 190(3): 501-8.
[http://dx.doi.org/10.1002/cne.901900307] [PMID: 6771304]

[17]   Molday RS, Hicks D, Molday L. Peripherin. A rim-specific membrane protein of rod outer segment discs. Invest Ophthalmol Vis Sci 1987; 28(1): 50-61.
[PMID: 2433249]

[18]   Wrigley JD, Ahmed T, Nevett CL, Findlay JB. Peripherin/rds influences membrane vesicle morphology. Implications for retinopathies. J Biol Chem 2000; 275(18): 13191-4.
[http://dx.doi.org/10.1074/jbc.C900853199] [PMID: 10747861]

[19]   Khattree N, Ritter LM, Goldberg AF. Membrane curvature generation by a C-terminal amphipathic helix in peripherin-2/rds, a tetraspanin required for photoreceptor sensory cilium morphogenesis. J Cell Sci 2013; 126(Pt 20): 4659-70.
[http://dx.doi.org/10.1242/jcs.126888] [PMID: 23886945]

[20]   Kevany BM, Tsybovsky Y, Campuzano ID, Schnier PD, Engel A, Palczewski K. Structural and functional analysis of the native peripherin-ROM1 complex isolated from photoreceptor cells. J Biol Chem 2013; 288(51): 36272-84.
[http://dx.doi.org/10.1074/jbc.M113.520700] [PMID: 24196967]

[21]   Travis GH, Sutcliffe JG, Bok D. The retinal degeneration slow (rds) gene product is a photoreceptor disc membrane-associated glycoprotein. Neuron 1991; 6(1): 61-70.
[http://dx.doi.org/10.1016/0896-6273(91)90122-G] [PMID: 1986774]

[22]   Wrigley JD, Nevett CL, Findlay JB. Topological analysis of peripherin/rds and abnormal glycosylation of the pathogenic Pro216-->Leu mutation. Biochem J 2002; 368(Pt 2): 649-55.

[http://dx.doi.org/10.1042/bj20020547] [PMID: 12207562]

[23] Conley SM, Stuck MW, Naash MI. Structural and functional relationships between photoreceptor tetraspanins and other superfamily members. Cell Mol Life Sci 2012; 69(7): 1035-47.
[http://dx.doi.org/10.1007/s00018-011-0736-0] [PMID: 21655915]

[24] Boesze-Battaglia K, Song H, Sokolov M, *et al.* The tetraspanin protein peripherin-2 forms a complex with melanoregulin, a putative membrane fusion regulator. Biochemistry 2007; 46(5): 1256-72.
[http://dx.doi.org/10.1021/bi061466i] [PMID: 17260955]

[25] Boesze-Battaglia K, Stefano FP, Fitzgerald C, Muller-Weeks S. ROM-1 potentiates photoreceptor specific membrane fusion processes. Exp Eye Res 2007; 84(1): 22-31.
[http://dx.doi.org/10.1016/j.exer.2006.08.010] [PMID: 17055485]

[26] Ritter LM, Boesze-Battaglia K, Tam BM, *et al.* Uncoupling of photoreceptor peripherin/rds fusogenic activity from biosynthesis, subunit assembly, and targeting: a potential mechanism for pathogenic effects. J Biol Chem 2004; 279(38): 39958-67.
[http://dx.doi.org/10.1074/jbc.M403943200] [PMID: 15252042]

[27] Poetsch A, Molday LL, Molday RS. The cGMP-gated channel and related glutamic acid-rich proteins interact with peripherin-2 at the rim region of rod photoreceptor disc membranes. J Biol Chem 2001; 276(51): 48009-16.
[http://dx.doi.org/10.1074/jbc.M108941200] [PMID: 11641407]

[28] Tam BM, Moritz OL, Papermaster DS. The C terminus of peripherin/rds participates in rod outer segment targeting and alignment of disk incisures. Mol Biol Cell 2004; 15(4): 2027-37.
[http://dx.doi.org/10.1091/mbc.E03-09-0650] [PMID: 14767063]

[29] Lapointe R, Yeagle PL, Gretzula CL, Boesze-Battaglia K. Peripherin-2: an intracellular analogy to viral fusion proteins. Biochemistry (Mosc) 2007; 46(12): 3605-13.
[http://dx.doi.org/10.1021/bi061820c]

[30] Salinas RY, Baker SA, Gospe SM III, Arshavsky VY. A single valine residue plays an essential role in peripherin/rds targeting to photoreceptor outer segments. PLoS One 2013; 8(1): e54292.
[http://dx.doi.org/10.1371/journal.pone.0054292] [PMID: 23342122]

[31] Conley SM, Ding XQ, Naash MI. RDS in cones does not interact with the beta subunit of the cyclic nucleotide gated channel. Adv Exp Med Biol 2010; 664: 63-70.
[http://dx.doi.org/10.1007/978-1-4419-1399-9_8] [PMID: 20238003]

[32] Boesze-Battaglia K, Lamba OP, Napoli AA Jr, Sinha S, Guo Y. Fusion between retinal rod outer segment membranes and model membranes: a role for photoreceptor peripherin/rds. Biochemistry 1998; 37(26): 9477-87.
[http://dx.doi.org/10.1021/bi980173p] [PMID: 9649331]

[33] Goldberg AF, Molday RS. Subunit composition of the peripherin/rds-rom-1 disk rim complex from rod photoreceptors: hydrodynamic evidence for a tetrameric quaternary structure. Biochemistry 1996; 35(19): 6144-9.
[http://dx.doi.org/10.1021/bi960259n] [PMID: 8634257]

[34] Clarke G, Goldberg AF, Vidgen D, *et al.* Rom-1 is required for rod photoreceptor viability and the regulation of disk morphogenesis. Nat Genet 2000; 25(1): 67-73.
[http://dx.doi.org/10.1038/75621] [PMID: 10802659]

[35] Loewen CJ, Molday RS. Disulfide-mediated oligomerization of Peripherin/Rds and Rom-1 in photoreceptor disk membranes. Implications for photoreceptor outer segment morphogenesis and degeneration. J Biol Chem 2000; 275(8): 5370-8.
[http://dx.doi.org/10.1074/jbc.275.8.5370] [PMID: 10681511]

[36] Bascom RA, Manara S, Collins L, Molday RS, Kalnins VI, McInnes RR. Cloning of the cDNA for a novel photoreceptor membrane protein (rom-1) identifies a disk rim protein family implicated in human retinopathies. Neuron 1992; 8(6): 1171-84.

[http://dx.doi.org/10.1016/0896-6273(92)90137-3] [PMID: 1610568]

[37]   Goldberg AF, Ritter LM, Khattree N, *et al.* An intramembrane glutamic acid governs peripherin/rds function for photoreceptor disk morphogenesis. Invest Ophthalmol Vis Sci 2007; 48(7): 2975-86.
       [http://dx.doi.org/10.1167/iovs.07-0049] [PMID: 17591862]

[38]   Kedzierski W, Nusinowitz S, Birch D, *et al.* Deficiency of rds/peripherin causes photoreceptor death in mouse models of digenic and dominant retinitis pigmentosa. Proc Natl Acad Sci USA 2001; 98(14): 7718-23.
       [http://dx.doi.org/10.1073/pnas.141124198] [PMID: 11427722]

[39]   Kedzierski W, Weng J, Travis GH. Analysis of the rds/peripherin.rom1 complex in transgenic photoreceptors that express a chimeric protein. J Biol Chem 1999; 274(41): 29181-7.
       [http://dx.doi.org/10.1074/jbc.274.41.29181] [PMID: 10506174]

[40]   Goldberg AF, Moritz OL, Molday RS. Heterologous expression of photoreceptor peripherin/rds and Rom-1 in COS-1 cells: assembly, interactions, and localization of multisubunit complexes. Biochemistry 1995; 34(43): 14213-9.
       [http://dx.doi.org/10.1021/bi00043a028] [PMID: 7578020]

[41]   Boesze-Battaglia K, Dispoto J, Kahoe MA. Association of a photoreceptor-specific tetraspanin protein, ROM-1, with triton X-100-resistant membrane rafts from rod outer segment disk membranes. J Biol Chem 2002; 277(44): 41843-9.
       [http://dx.doi.org/10.1074/jbc.M207111200] [PMID: 12196538]

[42]   Goldberg AF, Loewen CJ, Molday RS. Cysteine residues of photoreceptor peripherin/rds: role in subunit assembly and autosomal dominant retinitis pigmentosa. Biochemistry 1998; 37(2): 680-5.
       [http://dx.doi.org/10.1021/bi972036i] [PMID: 9425091]

[43]   Chakraborty D, Ding XQ, Fliesler SJ, Naash MI. Outer segment oligomerization of Rds: evidence from mouse models and subcellular fractionation. Biochemistry 2008; 47(4): 1144-56.
       [http://dx.doi.org/10.1021/bi701807c] [PMID: 18171083]

[44]   Chakraborty D, Conley SM, Stuck MW, Naash MI. Differences in RDS trafficking, assembly and function in cones *versus* rods: insights from studies of C150S-RDS. Hum Mol Genet 2010; 19(24): 4799-812.
       [http://dx.doi.org/10.1093/hmg/ddq410] [PMID: 20858597]

[45]   Chakraborty D, Conley SM, Fliesler SJ, Naash MI. The function of oligomerization-incompetent RDS in rods. Adv Exp Med Biol 2010; 664: 39-46.
       [http://dx.doi.org/10.1007/978-1-4419-1399-9_5] [PMID: 20238000]

[46]   Chakraborty D, Ding XQ, Conley SM, Fliesler SJ, Naash MI. Differential requirements for retinal degeneration slow intermolecular disulfide-linked oligomerization in rods *versus* cones. Hum Mol Genet 2009; 18(5): 797-808.
       [http://dx.doi.org/10.1093/hmg/ddn406] [PMID: 19050038]

[47]   Kajiwara K, Berson EL, Dryja TP. Digenic retinitis pigmentosa due to mutations at the unlinked peripherin/RDS and ROM1 loci. Science 1994; 264(5165): 1604-8.
       [http://dx.doi.org/10.1126/science.8202715] [PMID: 8202715]

[48]   Ma J, Norton JC, Allen AC, *et al.* Retinal degeneration slow (rds) in mouse results from simple insertion of a t haplotype-specific element into protein-coding exon II. Genomics 1995; 28(2): 212-9.
       [http://dx.doi.org/10.1006/geno.1995.1133] [PMID: 8530028]

[49]   Cheng T, Peachey NS, Li S, Goto Y, Cao Y, Naash MI. The effect of peripherin/rds haploinsufficiency on rod and cone photoreceptors. J Neurosci 1997; 17(21): 8118-28.
       [PMID: 9334387]

[50]   Stricker HM, Ding XQ, Quiambao A, Fliesler SJ, Naash MI. The Cys214-->Ser mutation in peripherin/rds causes a loss-of-function phenotype in transgenic mice. Biochem J 2005; 388(Pt 2): 605-13.

[http://dx.doi.org/10.1042/BJ20041960] [PMID: 15656787]

[51]   Kedzierski W, Lloyd M, Birch DG, Bok D, Travis GH. Generation and analysis of transgenic mice expressing P216L-substituted rds/peripherin in rod photoreceptors. Invest Ophthalmol Vis Sci 1997; 38(2): 498-509.
[PMID: 9040483]

[52]   Nour M, Ding XQ, Stricker H, Fliesler SJ, Naash MI. Modulating expression of peripherin/rds in transgenic mice: critical levels and the effect of overexpression. Invest Ophthalmol Vis Sci 2004; 45(8): 2514-21.
[http://dx.doi.org/10.1167/iovs.04-0065] [PMID: 15277471]

[53]   Farjo R, Fliesler SJ, Naash MI. Effect of Rds abundance on cone outer segment morphogenesis, photoreceptor gene expression, and outer limiting membrane integrity. J Comp Neurol 2007; 504(6): 619-30.
[http://dx.doi.org/10.1002/cne.21476] [PMID: 17722028]

[54]   Farjo R, Skaggs JS, Nagel BA, *et al.* Retention of function without normal disc morphogenesis occurs in cone but not rod photoreceptors. J Cell Biol 2006; 173(1): 59-68.
[http://dx.doi.org/10.1083/jcb.200509036] [PMID: 16585269]

[55]   Strauss O. The retinal pigment epithelium in visual function. Physiol Rev 2005; 85(3): 845-81.
[http://dx.doi.org/10.1152/physrev.00021.2004] [PMID: 15987797]

[56]   Stuck MW, Conley SM, Naash MI. The Y141C knockin mutation in RDS leads to complex phenotypes in the mouse. Hum Mol Genet 2014; 23(23): 6260-74.
[http://dx.doi.org/10.1093/hmg/ddu345] [PMID: 25001182]

[57]   Francis PJ, Schultz DW, Gregory AM, *et al.* Genetic and phenotypic heterogeneity in pattern dystrophy. Br J Ophthalmol 2005; 89(9): 1115-9.
[http://dx.doi.org/10.1136/bjo.2004.062695] [PMID: 16113362]

[58]   Duncan JL, Talcott KE, Ratnam K, *et al.* Cone structure in retinal degeneration associated with mutations in the peripherin/RDS gene. Invest Ophthalmol Vis Sci 2011; 52(3): 1557-66.
[http://dx.doi.org/10.1167/iovs.10-6549] [PMID: 21071739]

[59]   Wroblewski JJ, Wells JA III, Eckstein A, *et al.* Macular dystrophy associated with mutations at codon 172 in the human retinal degeneration slow gene. Ophthalmology 1994; 101(1): 12-22.
[http://dx.doi.org/10.1016/S0161-6420(94)31377-7] [PMID: 8302543]

[60]   Michaelides M, Holder GE, Bradshaw K, Hunt DM, Moore AT. Cone-rod dystrophy, intrafamilial variability, and incomplete penetrance associated with the R172W mutation in the peripherin/RDS gene. Ophthalmology 2005; 112(9): 1592-8.
[http://dx.doi.org/10.1016/j.ophtha.2005.04.004] [PMID: 16019073]

[61]   Poloschek CM, Bach M, Lagrèze WA, *et al.* ABCA4 and ROM1: implications for modification of the PRPH2-associated macular dystrophy phenotype. Invest Ophthalmol Vis Sci 2010; 51(8): 4253-65.
[http://dx.doi.org/10.1167/iovs.09-4655] [PMID: 20335603]

[62]   Leroy BP, Kailasanathan A, De Laey JJ, Black GC, Manson FD. Intrafamilial phenotypic variability in families with RDS mutations: exclusion of ROM1 as a genetic modifier for those with retinitis pigmentosa. Br J Ophthalmol 2007; 91(1): 89-93.
[http://dx.doi.org/10.1136/bjo.2006.101915] [PMID: 16916875]

[63]   Conley SM, Stuck MW, Burnett JL, *et al.* Insights into the mechanisms of macular degeneration associated with the R172W mutation in RDS. Hum Mol Genet 2014; 23(12): 3102-14.
[http://dx.doi.org/10.1093/hmg/ddu014] [PMID: 24463884]

[64]   Conley SM, Stricker HM, Naash MI. Biochemical analysis of phenotypic diversity associated with mutations in codon 244 of the retinal degeneration slow gene. Biochemistry 2010; 49(5): 905-11.
[http://dx.doi.org/10.1021/bi901622w] [PMID: 20055437]

[65]   Ding XQ, Nour M, Ritter LM, Goldberg AF, Fliesler SJ, Naash MI. The R172W mutation in

peripherin/rds causes a cone-rod dystrophy in transgenic mice. Hum Mol Genet 2004; 13(18): 2075-87.
[http://dx.doi.org/10.1093/hmg/ddh211] [PMID: 15254014]

[66]   Kikawa E, Nakazawa M, Chida Y, Shiono T, Tamai M. A novel mutation (Asn244Lys) in the peripherin/RDS gene causing autosomal dominant retinitis pigmentosa associated with bull's-eye maculopathy detected by nonradioisotopic SSCP. Genomics 1994; 20(1): 137-9.
[http://dx.doi.org/10.1006/geno.1994.1142] [PMID: 8020945]

[67]   Nakazawa M, Kikawa E, Chida Y, Tamai M. Asn244His mutation of the peripherin/RDS gene causing autosomal dominant cone-rod degeneration. Hum Mol Genet 1994; 3(7): 1195-6.
[http://dx.doi.org/10.1093/hmg/3.7.1195] [PMID: 7981698]

[68]   Conley S, Nour M, Fliesler SJ, Naash MI. Late-onset cone photoreceptor degeneration induced by R172W mutation in Rds and partial rescue by gene supplementation. Invest Ophthalmol Vis Sci 2007; 48(12): 5397-407.
[http://dx.doi.org/10.1167/iovs.07-0663] [PMID: 18055786]

[69]   Cai X, Conley SM, Naash MI. Gene therapy in the Retinal Degeneration Slow model of retinitis pigmentosa. Adv Exp Med Biol 2010; 664: 611-9.
[http://dx.doi.org/10.1007/978-1-4419-1399-9_70] [PMID: 20238065]

[70]   Cai X, Conley SM, Nash Z, Fliesler SJ, Cooper MJ, Naash MI. Gene delivery to mitotic and postmitotic photoreceptors *via* compacted DNA nanoparticles results in improved phenotype in a mouse model of retinitis pigmentosa. FASEB J 2010; 24(4): 1178-91.
[http://dx.doi.org/10.1096/fj.09-139147] [PMID: 19952284]

[71]   Ali RR, Sarra GM, Stephens C, *et al.* Restoration of photoreceptor ultrastructure and function in retinal degeneration slow mice by gene therapy. Nat Genet 2000; 25(3): 306-10.
[http://dx.doi.org/10.1038/77068] [PMID: 10888879]

[72]   Sarra GM, Stephens C, de Alwis M, *et al.* Gene replacement therapy in the retinal degeneration slow (rds) mouse: the effect on retinal degeneration following partial transduction of the retina. Hum Mol Genet 2001; 10(21): 2353-61.
[http://dx.doi.org/10.1093/hmg/10.21.2353] [PMID: 11689482]

[73]   Thompson S, Blodi FR, Lee S, *et al.* Photoreceptor cells with profound structural deficits can support useful vision in mice. Invest Ophthalmol Vis Sci 2014; 55(3): 1859-66.
[http://dx.doi.org/10.1167/iovs.13-13661] [PMID: 24569582]

[74]   Liang FQ, Aleman TS, Dejneka NS, *et al.* Long-term protection of retinal structure but not function using RAAV.CNTF in animal models of retinitis pigmentosa. Mol Ther 2001; 4(5): 461-72.
[http://dx.doi.org/10.1006/mthe.2001.0473] [PMID: 11708883]

[75]   Cayouette M, Behn D, Sendtner M, Lachapelle P, Gravel C. Intraocular gene transfer of ciliary neurotrophic factor prevents death and increases responsiveness of rod photoreceptors in the retinal degeneration slow mouse. J Neurosci 1998; 18(22): 9282-93.
[PMID: 9801367]

[76]   Cayouette M, Smith SB, Becerra SP, Gravel C. Pigment epithelium-derived factor delays the death of photoreceptors in mouse models of inherited retinal degenerations. Neurobiol Dis 1999; 6(6): 523-32.
[http://dx.doi.org/10.1006/nbdi.1999.0263] [PMID: 10600408]

[77]   Eigeldinger-Berthou S, Meier C, Zulliger R, Lecaudé S, Enzmann V, Sarra GM. Rasagiline interferes with neurodegeneration in the Prph2/rds mouse. Retina 2012; 32(3): 617-28.
[http://dx.doi.org/10.1097/IAE.0b013e31821e2070] [PMID: 21878836]

CHAPTER 7

Rhodopsin-Regulated Grb14 Trafficking to Rod Outer Segments: Functional Role of Grb14 in Photoreceptors

Raju V.S. Rajala[*]

Departments of Ophthalmology, Physiology, and Cell Biology, University of Oklahoma Health Sciences Center, and Dean A. McGee Eye Institute, Oklahoma City, Oklahoma 73104, USA

Abstract: Growth factor receptor-bound protein 14 (Grb14) belongs to the Grb7 family. It is an adapter molecule, lacking any intrinsic enzyme activity, but mediates protein-protein and protein-lipid interactions. In photoreceptors, Grb14 undergoes a rhodopsin-dependent translocation from the inner segments to the outer segments. In photoreceptors, Grb14 undergoes a light-dependent tyrosine phosphorylation and protects the insulin receptor (IR) phosphorylation, which is neuroprotective. Outer-segment-localized Grb14 also modulates the activity of the cyclic nucleotide gated (CNG) chancel. Thus, Grb14 plays a key role in receiving signals from rhodopsin, and translocating to outer segments, where it regulates IR and CNG channel activities. The present study supports the idea that rhodopsin regulates non-canonical signaling pathways in photoreceptor cells.

Keywords: CNG channel, Grb14, Insulin receptor, PTP1B, Rhodopsin, Rod outer segments, Tyrosine phosphorylation.

INTRODUCTION

Signaling from tyrosine kinases is commonly facilitated by scaffold and adapter proteins, with domains, such as Src-homology-2 (SH2) and phosphotyrosine-binding (PTB), that bind precise phosphotyrosine sites and elements that selectively link to downstream targets that activate cytoplasmic pathways. Growth factor receptor-bound protein (Grb14) is an adapter protein that belongs to the Grb7 family, which includes Grb7 and Grb10 [1, 2]. All Grb7-family members have well-defined regions/domains of a proline-rich motif (PS/AIPNPFPEL), a Ras-associating (RA) domain, a Pleckstrin-homology (PH) domain, a "Between the PH and SH2 domain" (BPS) region, and a Src-homology (SH2) domain (Fig. **1**) [2].

[*] **Corresponding author Raju V.S. Rajala:** University of Oklahoma Health Sciences Center, and Dean McGee Eye Institute, Oklahoma City, Oklahoma, USA; Tel: 405 271 8255; E-mail: raju-rajala@ouhsc.edu

Hemant Khanna (Ed)

Decades ago, researchers observed a close resemblance between the RA and PH domains of Grb7 and a cell migration protein, Mig10, from *Caenorhabditis elegans* [3]. The Mig10 protein belongs to the MRL protein family [4, 5]. The most remarkable difference between the Grb7 and MRL proteins is the presence of the BPS domain and a C-terminal SH2 domain in the Grb7 family of proteins [4]. The Grb7 family of proteins has a unique BPS domain [1]. It has been shown that the insulin receptor (IR) associates with the BPS domain of Grb10 and Grb14 [6 - 8]. The PH domains of Grb7 [2] and Grb14 [6] interact with phosphoinositides; however, the protein-lipid interaction in cellular signaling is not fully understood. Through SH2 domains, several receptor tyrosine kinases and many signaling molecules can interact with Grb7, Grb10, and Grb14 [1]. These Grb7 family proteins have been shown to be localized mainly in the cytoplasm, and in certain cases have been observed in the plasma membrane, focal contacts, and mitochondria [2]. The phosphorylation on serine/threonine and tyrosine residues in Grb7, Grb10, and Grb14 has been observed. However, their functional significance has not been elucidated [2]. In this review, we describe Grb14's unique roles in rod photoreceptor cells.

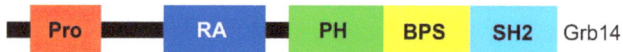

Fig. (1). Domain organization of Grb14. Pro, proline rich region, RA, ras-associating domain, PH, pleckstrin homology domain, BPS, between PH and SH2 domain, SH2, Src-homology region.

Grb14 Role in Insulin Receptor Signaling

Grb14 is a pseudo-substrate inhibitor of the IR [9], and negatively regulates IR signaling through inhibition of its kinase activity [8, 10]. The BPS domain of Grb14 interacts with the IR [8]. These observations were further supported by a genome-wide association study showing that reduced insulin sensitivity in patients with diabetes is strongly associated with single nucleotide polymorphisms in Grb14 [11]. These findings were further supported by research with Grb14 knockout mice, which showed improved glucose homeostasis and enhanced insulin signaling [12], confirming the negative role of Grb14 in insulin signaling. In myocardial tissues, Grb14 is important in the activation of the PI3K/Akt signaling pathway; Grb14 ablation has been shown to result in myocardial infarction [13]. IR signaling is essential for photoreceptor neuroprotection, and ablation of IR in rods leads to stress-induced photoreceptor degeneration, whereas ablation in cones results in cone degeneration without added stress [14, 15]. Interestingly, Grb14 is expressed in the retina, and it inhibits IR kinase activity *in vitro* [10]. However, Grb14 knockout mice exhibited reduced IR activation *in vivo* due to increased activity of protein tyrosine phosphatase 1B (PTP1B) [16]. Similarly, reduced activation of IR due to increased phosphatase activity has been observed in the liver tissues of Grb14 knockout mice [12]. In the retina, IR activation is light-dependent and is due to light-dependent inhibition of PTP1B activity [17]. The mechanism behind the light-induced activation of IR is light-dependent phosphorylation of Grb14 by a non-receptor tyrosine kinase, Src [16]. The phosphorylated Grb14 binds to PTP1B and inhibits its activity [16]. The non-phosphorylated form of Grb14 has a higher affinity for IR, whereas the phosphorylated form of Grb14 has a higher affinity for PTP1B [16]. The light-induced activation of IR, inhibition of PTP1B activity, activation of Src, and phosphorylation of Grb14 are mediated through a rhodopsin-dependent, G-protein coupled receptor [16]. Rhodopsin activation determines the state of Grb14 phosphorylation and IR-mediated neuroprotection *in vivo* [15, 16]). The mechanism of IR activation by Grb14 is described in Fig. (**2**). Mutations in the rhodopsin gene and mice that are unable to activate rhodopsin exhibit retinal degeneration due to the absence of Src activation, Grb14 phosphorylation, increased PTP1B activity, and subsequent inactivation of IR signaling [15, 16]. These findings suggest that activators of Src or inhibitors of PTP1B may be able to rescue the retinal degeneration phenotype.

Negative Regulatory Role of Grb14 on Insulin Receptor Signaling

Grb14 is an insulin receptor (IR)-interacting protein in the retina [3]. Interestingly, Grb14 is a pseudo-substrate inhibitor of IR [2] and inhibits IR tyrosine kinase activity. Consistent with these findings, a genome-wide association study demonstrated that single nucleotide polymorphisms at Grb14 are strongly associated with reduced insulin sensitivity in diabetic patients [4]. IR signaling is essential for photoreceptors, as deletion of IR [5] or proteins involved in the IR signaling pathway leads to both rod and cone degeneration [6, 7]. In addition to Grb14, IR signaling is also negatively regulated by protein tyrosine phosphatase, PTP1B [8]. Thus, the major question remains: how does the IR overcome inactivation by PTP1B and Grb14 in retinal neurons? This review primarily focuses on the intracellular localization and spatial and temporal regulation of Grb14 on IR signaling.

Light-Dependent Translocation of Grb14 in Rod Photoreceptor Cells

In dark-adapted retina, Grb14 is predominantly localized to photoreceptor inner segments [18]. Upon light-illumination, a certain portion of Grb14 translocates to the rod outer segments [18] (Fig. **3**). The binding of Grb14 to rod outer segment membranes is also light-dependent [18, 19]. This binding does not require transducin signaling, but requires the photobleaching of rhodopsin [18]. Grb14 is predominantly associated with the outer segment plasma membrane, but not the disc membranes [20]. In mice lacking rhodopsin photobleaching, Grb14 is localized to the outer segments in both dark- and light-adapted conditions [18]. In rod photoreceptor cells, three proteins, transducin, arrestin, and recoverin, which are involved in phototransduction, undergo light-dependent translocation [21, 22]. However, Grb14, which is not involved in phototransduction, still undergoes light-dependent translocation upon rhodopsin activation [18]. These studies suggest that rhodopsin can initiate a non-canonical signaling pathway in rod photoreceptor cells.

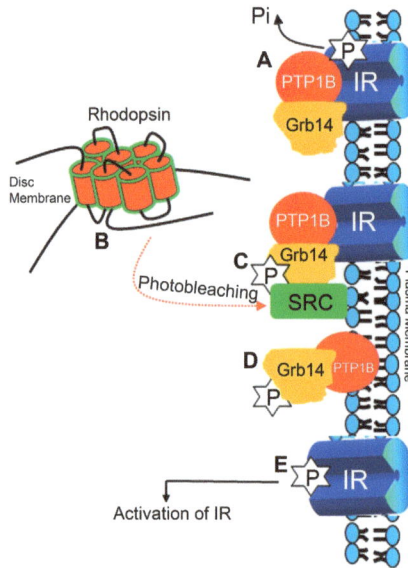

Fig. (2). Grb14 positively regulates the IR signaling pathway. The insulin receptor (IR) in the retina is constitutively phosphorylated (activation). Activation of IR is negatively regulated by PTP1B and Grb14. PTP1B directly dephosphorylates phosphate groups on the IR, while Grb14 directly binds to the active site of the IR and inactivates it (**A**). The IR overcomes the inactivation by both PTP1B and Grb14 through the photobleaching of rhodopsin (**B**) which activates a non-receptor tyrosine kinase, Src (**C**). Src phosphorylates Grb14, and the phosphorylated Grb14 binds to the active site of the PTP1B and inactivates it (**D**), thereby relieving the inhibitory constrains on the IR (**E**). Thus, the IR becomes active, and regulates the downstream effector cascade, which provides neuroprotection to the retina. IR, insulin receptor; P, phosphorylation; Pi, inorganic phosphate; Grb14, growth factor receptor bound-protein 14; SRC, non-receptor tyrosine kinase Src; PTP1B, protein tyrosine phosphatase 1B.

Cross-Talk between Rhodopsin Activation and Grb14 Signaling

Grb14 was originally identified as an IR interacting protein in the retina [10, 23]. In IR knockout mice, the light-dependent translocation of Grb14 to outer segments and its binding to rod outer segment membranes is unaffected [18]. These findings suggest that Grb14 may have other targets in rod outer segments, in addition to the IR. Protein-interaction studies show that Grb14 associates with photoreceptor-specific cyclic-nucleotide-gated channel alpha subunit (CNGA1), and decreases its affinity for cGMP [19]. This interaction is mediated through the

RA-domain of Grb14 with the C-terminal region of the CNGA1 subunit [19, 20, 24]. In dark-adapted photoreceptor cells, a high concentration of cGMP binds to the CNG channel and facilitates its opening [25]. Upon on light-adaptation through rhodopsin activation, the GTP-bound G-protein transducin alpha subunit binds to the inhibitory subunit of cGMP-phosphodiesterase (cGMP-PDE) and activates the PDE, which hydrolyzes the cGMP to GMP, thereby closing the channel. Interestingly, under light-adapted conditions, the channel remains open in Grb14 knockout mice [19]. Ablation of Grb14 also produced an increase in channel affinity for cGMP in rod cells [26]. Suction-electrode recordings from single Grb14-knockout mouse rods also show a significant decrease in the limiting time constant, indicating the modulation of the rate of inactivation of cGMP-PDE6, rather than a direct effect on the channel [26]. This observation that rhodopsin photobleaching activates the translocation of Grb14 to outer segments, which bind to CNGA1 and modulate its activity, is novel. Outside of photoreceptors, tyrosine kinase signaling is modulated by G-protein-coupled receptors [27, 28]. Our studies suggest that rhodopsin activates tyrosine kinases and adapter proteins involved in tyrosine kinase signaling in photoreceptor cells.

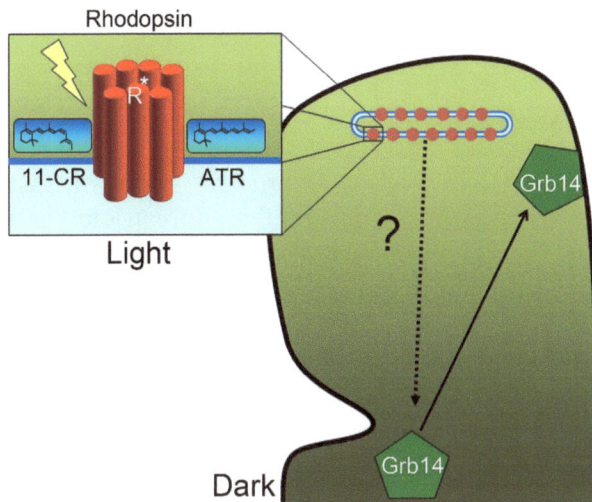

Fig. (3). Light-dependent translocation of Grb14. In the dark, Grb14 localized to rod inner segments. Upon light activation, through photobleaching of rhodopsin, Grb14 moves to outer segments by a yet-to-be-determined unknown mechanism. 11-CR, 11-*cis*-retinal, ATR, all-*trans* retinal.

CONCLUDING REMARKS

In summary, the findings suggest that intracellular localization of Grb14 is necessary to spatially and temporally control insulin signaling and cyclic nucleotide-gated channel modulation. Further, activators of Grb14 phosphorylation may have the therapeutic potential to protect the dying retinal neurons in retinal degenerative diseases

LIST OF ABBREVIATIONS

Grb14   Growth factor receptor-bound protein 14

ROS   Rod outer segments

PTP1B   Protein tyrosine phosphatase 1B

IR   Insulin receptor

Rpe   Retinal pigment epithelium

Pro   Proline-rich region

RA   Ras-associating domain

PH   Pleckstrin-homology domain

BPS   Between the PH and SH2 domain

SH2   Src-homology domain

CNG   Cyclic nucleotide-gated channel

CONFLICT OF INTEREST

The author (editor) declares no conflict of interest, financial or otherwise.

ACKNOWLEDGEMENTS

This study was supported by grants from the National Institutes of Health (EY016507, EY00871, and EY021725), and an unrestricted grant from Research to Prevent Blindness, Inc. to the Department of Ophthalmology.

REFERENCES

[1]   Daly RJ. The Grb7 family of signalling proteins. Cell Signal 1998; 10(9): 613-8.
[http://dx.doi.org/10.1016/S0898-6568(98)00022-9] [PMID: 9794242]

[2]   Han DC, Shen TL, Guan JL. The Grb7 family proteins: structure, interactions with other signaling molecules and potential cellular functions. Oncogene 2001; 20(44): 6315-21.
[http://dx.doi.org/10.1038/sj.onc.1204775] [PMID: 11607834]

[3]   Manser J, Roonprapunt C, Margolis B. C. elegans cell migration gene mig-10 shares similarities with a family of SH2 domain proteins and acts cell nonautonomously in excretory canal development. Dev Biol 1997; 184(1): 150-64.
[http://dx.doi.org/10.1006/dbio.1997.8516] [PMID: 9142991]

[4]   Holt LJ, Daly RJ. Adapter protein connections: the MRL and Grb7 protein families. Growth Factors 2005; 23(3): 193-201.
[http://dx.doi.org/10.1080/08977190500196267] [PMID: 16243711]

[5]   Legg JA, Machesky LM. MRL proteins: leading Ena/VASP to Ras GTPases. Nat Cell Biol 2004; 6(11): 1015-7.
[http://dx.doi.org/10.1038/ncb1104-1015] [PMID: 15516992]

[6]   Rajala RV, Chan MD, Rajala A. Lipid-protein interactions of growth factor receptor-bound protein 14 in insulin receptor signaling. Biochemistry 2005; 44(47): 15461-71.
[http://dx.doi.org/10.1021/bi0513148] [PMID: 16300394]

[7]   Stein EG, Gustafson TA, Hubbard SR. The BPS domain of Grb10 inhibits the catalytic activity of the insulin and IGF1 receptors. FEBS Lett 2001; 493(2-3): 106-11.
[http://dx.doi.org/10.1016/S0014-5793(01)02282-7] [PMID: 11287005]

[8]   Béréziat V, Kasus-Jacobi A, Perdereau D, Cariou B, Girard J, Burnol AF. Inhibition of insulin receptor catalytic activity by the molecular adapter Grb14. J Biol Chem 2002; 277(7): 4845-52.
[http://dx.doi.org/10.1074/jbc.M106574200] [PMID: 11726652]

[9]   Depetris RS, Hu J, Gimpelevich I, Holt LJ, Daly RJ, Hubbard SR. Structural basis for inhibition of the insulin receptor by the adaptor protein Grb14. Mol Cell 2005; 20(2): 325-33.
[http://dx.doi.org/10.1016/j.molcel.2005.09.001] [PMID: 16246733]

[10]   Rajala RV, Chan MD. Identification of a NPXY motif in growth factor receptor-bound protein 14 (Grb14) and its interaction with the phosphotyrosine-binding (PTB) domain of IRS-1. Biochemistry 2005; 44(22): 7929-35.
[http://dx.doi.org/10.1021/bi0500271] [PMID: 15924411]

[11]   Kooner JS, Saleheen D, Sim X, *et al.* Genome-wide association study in individuals of South Asian ancestry identifies six new type 2 diabetes susceptibility loci. Nat Genet 2011; 43(10): 984-9.
[http://dx.doi.org/10.1038/ng.921] [PMID: 21874001]

[12]   Cooney GJ, Lyons RJ, Crew AJ, *et al.* Improved glucose homeostasis and enhanced insulin signalling in Grb14-deficient mice. EMBO J 2004; 23(3): 582-93.
[http://dx.doi.org/10.1038/sj.emboj.7600082] [PMID: 14749734]

[13]   Lin RC, Weeks KL, Gao XM, *et al.* PI3K(p110 alpha) protects against myocardial infarction-induced heart failure: identification of PI3K-regulated miRNA and mRNA. Arterioscler Thromb Vasc Biol 2010; 30(4): 724-32.
[http://dx.doi.org/10.1161/ATVBAHA.109.201988] [PMID: 20237330]

[14]   Rajala A, Tanito M, Le YZ, Kahn CR, Rajala RV. Loss of neuroprotective survival signal in mice lacking insulin receptor gene in rod photoreceptor cells. J Biol Chem 2008; 283(28): 19781-92.
[http://dx.doi.org/10.1074/jbc.M802374200] [PMID: 18480052]

[15]   Rajala A, Wang Y, Rajala RV. Activation of oncogenic tyrosine kinase signaling promotes insulin receptor-mediated cone photoreceptor survival. Oncotarget 2016; 7(30): 46924-42.
[PMID: 27391439]

[16]   Basavarajappa DK, Gupta VK, Dighe R, Rajala A, Rajala RV. Phosphorylated Grb14 is an endogenous inhibitor of retinal protein tyrosine phosphatase 1B, and light-dependent activation of Src phosphorylates Grb14. Mol Cell Biol 2011; 31(19): 3975-87.
[http://dx.doi.org/10.1128/MCB.05659-11] [PMID: 21791607]

[17]   Rajala RV, Tanito M, Neel BG, Rajala A. Enhanced retinal insulin receptor-activated neuroprotective survival signal in mice lacking the protein-tyrosine phosphatase-1B gene. J Biol Chem 2010; 285(12): 8894-904.
[http://dx.doi.org/10.1074/jbc.M109.070854] [PMID: 20061388]

[18]   Rajala A, Daly RJ, Tanito M, *et al.* Growth factor receptor-bound protein 14 undergoes light-dependent intracellular translocation in rod photoreceptors: functional role in retinal insulin receptor activation. Biochemistry 2009; 48(24): 5563-72.
[http://dx.doi.org/10.1021/bi9000062] [PMID: 19438210]

[19]   Gupta VK, Rajala A, Daly RJ, Rajala RV. Growth factor receptor-bound protein 14: a new modulator of photoreceptor-specific cyclic-nucleotide-gated channel. EMBO Rep 2010; 11(11): 861-7.
[http://dx.doi.org/10.1038/embor.2010.142] [PMID: 20890309]

[20]   Rajala RV, Rajala A, Gupta VK. Conservation and divergence of Grb7 family of Ras-binding

domains. Protein Cell 2012; 3(1): 60-70.
[http://dx.doi.org/10.1007/s13238-012-2001-1] [PMID: 22271596]

[21]   Calvert PD, Strissel KJ, Schiesser WE, Pugh EN Jr, Arshavsky VY. Light-driven translocation of signaling proteins in vertebrate photoreceptors. Trends Cell Biol 2006; 16(11): 560-8.
[http://dx.doi.org/10.1016/j.tcb.2006.09.001] [PMID: 16996267]

[22]   Strissel KJ, Lishko PV, Trieu LH, Kennedy MJ, Hurley JB, Arshavsky VY. Recoverin undergoes light-dependent intracellular translocation in rod photoreceptors. J Biol Chem 2005; 280(32): 29250-5.
[http://dx.doi.org/10.1074/jbc.M501789200] [PMID: 15961391]

[23]   Kasus-Jacobi A, Perdereau D, Auzan C, *et al.* Identification of the rat adapter Grb14 as an inhibitor of insulin actions. J Biol Chem 1998; 273(40): 26026-35.
[http://dx.doi.org/10.1074/jbc.273.40.26026] [PMID: 9748281]

[24]   Gupta VK, Rajala A, Rodgers KK, Rajala RV. Mechanism involved in the modulation of photoreceptor-specific cyclic nucleotidegated channel by the tyrosine kinase adapter protein Grb14. Protein Cell 2011; 2(11): 906-17.
[http://dx.doi.org/10.1007/s13238-011-1115-1] [PMID: 22180090]

[25]   Kaupp UB, Seifert R. Cyclic nucleotide-gated ion channels. Physiol Rev 2002; 82(3): 769-824.
[http://dx.doi.org/10.1152/physrev.00008.2002] [PMID: 12087135]

[26]   Woodruff ML, Rajala A, Fain GL, Rajala RV. Modulation of mouse rod photoreceptor responses by Grb14 protein. J Biol Chem 2014; 289(1): 358-64.
[http://dx.doi.org/10.1074/jbc.M113.517045] [PMID: 24273167]

[27]   Luttrell LM, van Biesen T, Hawes BE, *et al.* G-protein-coupled receptors and their regulation: activation of the MAP kinase signaling pathway by G-protein-coupled receptors. Adv Second Messenger Phosphoprotein Res 1997; 31: 263-77.
[http://dx.doi.org/10.1016/S1040-7952(97)80024-9] [PMID: 9344257]

[28]   Luttrell LM, Daaka Y, Lefkowitz RJ. Regulation of tyrosine kinase cascades by G-protein-coupled receptors. Curr Opin Cell Biol 1999; 11(2): 177-83.
[http://dx.doi.org/10.1016/S0955-0674(99)80023-4] [PMID: 10209148]

CHAPTER 8

Cellular Mechanisms of Cone Defects in Cyclic Nucleotide-Gated Channel Deficiency

Xi-Qin Ding[1,*], Hongwei Ma[1], Martin Biel[2] and Stylianos Michalakis[2]

[1] *Department of Cell Biology, University of Oklahoma Health Sciences Center, Oklahoma City, Oklahoma, USA*

[2] *Center for Integrated Protein Science Munich (CIPSM) and Department of Pharmacy - Center for Drug Research, Ludwig-Maximilians-Universität München, Munich, Germany*

Abstract: The cone photoreceptor-specific cyclic nucleotide-gated (CNG) channel is indispensable for cone function. Cones are essential for daylight vision and visual acuity. Mutations in the *CNGA3* and *CNGB3* genes are associated with achromatopsia, cone degeneration, and early-onset macular degeneration, and account for 80-85% of Achromatopsia cases. Patients with CNG channel defects exhibit cone dysfunction and progressive degeneration of cones, as revealed by electrophysiological recordings, psychophysical testing, and morphological examinations. The cellular events and underlying mechanisms of CNG channel deficiency have been explored using mouse models. In this review, we have summarized our current understanding of the modes of cone defects due to CNG channel deficiency.

Keywords: Apoptosis, cGMP, CNG channel, Cone, Endoplasmic reticulum, Mitochondrion, Photoreceptor, PKG, Retina.

INTRODUCTION

The photoreceptor cyclic nucleotide-gated (CNG) channels are located at the plasma membrane of the outer segments and are essential for phototransduction [1 - 4]. In darkness/dim light, binding of the channel ligand cyclic guanosine monophosphate (cGMP) activates CNG channels, allowing a steady depolarizing cation current, mostly mediated by Ca^{2+} and Na^+, to flow into the outer segment. Light induces hydrolysis of cGMP by the phosphodiesterase PDE6, resulting in channel closure and membrane hyperpolarization [1, 5, 6]. Interestingly, the light sensitivity, cGMP sensitivity, Ca^{2+} permeability, structural features, and functional modulation are profoundly different between rod and cone CNG channels [1, 4].

---
[*] **Corresponding author Xi-Qin Ding:** Department of Cell Biology, University of Oklahoma Health Sciences Center, 940 Stanton L. Young Blvd., BMSB 553, Oklahoma City, Oklahoma 73104, USA; Tel: (405) 271-8001; Ext: 47966; Fax: (405) 271-3548; E-mail: xi-qin-ding@ouhsc.edu

The CNG channel is the only source of Ca^{2+} influx into the outer segments. Therefore, this channel is important for intracellular Ca^{2+} homeostasis, which controls light response, cellular calcium signaling, and cGMP production. Structurally, the CNG channels are members of the pore-loop cation channel super family. They share a structural domain with hyperpolarization-activated cyclic nucleotide-gated (HCN) channels and K^+ channels [6 - 8]. The channel is composed of two subunits, the A and B subunits. The rod channel is composed of CNGA1/CNGB1 and the cone channel has CNGA3/CNGB3. Heterologous expression studies showed that the A subunits form the ion-conducting moiety, while the B subunits act as modulators [9 - 11]. Mutations in photoreceptor CNG channels are found in inherited retinal degenerative diseases [12 - 19].

Mutations in Cone CNG Channel Subunits and Human Cone Diseases

The human genes for CNGA3 and CNGB3 are located in 2q11.2 and 8q21-q22, respectively. Mutations in *CNGA3* and *CNGB3* have been identified in human patients with achromatopsia or rod monochromatism, cone-rod dystrophies, and early-onset macular degeneration [15 - 18]. *CNGA3* mutations were also identified in patients with Leber's congenital amaurosis [20]. To date, about 141 mutations in *CNGA3* and 63 mutations in *CNGB3* have been reported (www.hgmd.cf.ac.uk); these mutations are found in 80-85% of all achromatopsia [16, 17, 21 - 25]. As achromatopsia is primarily caused due to defects in the channel subunits, it is also called a "channelopathy" [26]. Achromatopsia is a severe retinal disorder with a prevalence of approximately 1 in 33,000 individuals. The patients report inability to distinguish colors, reduced visual acuity, photophobia/hemeralopia, and pendular nystagmus. Some patients also exhibit paradoxical pupillary constriction when transitioned from light to dark (Flynn phenomenon) [27]. Electroretinography (ERG) analysis revealed unmeasurable cone function and normal or abnormal rod function [18, 24, 28, 29]. Optical coherence tomography (OCT) [30 - 37] and adaptive optics scanning light ophthalmoscopy (AOSLO) [38, 39] studies have established cone loss in patients with achromatopsia associated with CNG channel mutations. Due to a founder effect, the *CNGB3* mutations are present in increased frequency in the Pingelapese population of the Pacific Islands [40].

Interestingly, patient population studies revealed some epidemiological features. Most achromatopsia cases in European populations arise from mutations in the CNGB3 subunit [18, 19, 21, 41], while mutations in CNGA3 are the leading cause of the disease among Asian populations [22 - 24, 42 - 46]. CNGA3 is the primary subunit, forming the ion-conducting unit. Heterologous expression studies showed that majority of *CNGA3* mutations are loss of function alleles [47 - 57]. Most disease-causing CNGB3 mutations are amino acid substitutions. However, the frame shift mutation, Thr383fsx, occurs most frequently and accounts for >80% of all *CNGB3* alleles [21, 41, 58, 59]. As the mutation truncates the pore and the C-terminal cytoplasmic domain, it is considered a null mutation. In addition, mutations in CNGA3 and CNGB3 have been found in sheep [60] and dog breeding [61 - 63] models of day blindness, respectively.

No treatment currently exists for CNG channelopathy. Gene therapy has shown promise for phenotype corrections [26]. Successful functional and structural rescue has been demonstrated following gene therapy in *Cnga3*$^{-/-}$ and *Cngb3*$^{-/-}$ mice and in canine models of CNGB3 mutations [61, 64 - 67]. Recently, the ciliary neurotrophic factor (CNTF) was shown to induce transient photoreceptor deconstruction and enhance cone functional rescue in canine models of CNGB3 deficiency [68], but the effect was not supported in human clinical trials [69].

Cone Defects in Mouse Models of CNG Channel Deficiency

The retinal phenotype of CNG channel deficiency has been examined in mouse models. *Cnga3*$^{-/-}$ and *Cngb3*$^{-/-}$ mice show reduced cone function and progressive cone degeneration [70 - 74]. As models of achromatopsia, these mouse lines have been used in studies of cone structure and function [71, 72], cone opsin plasma membrane targeting [70], retinal synaptic plasticity [74 - 76], visual acuity [72, 77], regulation of the channel subunit expression [72], mechanisms of cone degeneration [78], and gene replacement therapy [64 - 66]. Because cones comprise only 2-3% of the total photoreceptor population in the wild-type mouse retina, identification of the cellular alterations and biochemical events in CNG channel-deficient mice is challenging. To overcome this limitation and to better model the pathology in the cone-rich fovea-macular region of the human retina, *Cnga3*$^{-/-}$ and *Cngb3*$^{-/-}$ mice have been crossed with the *Nrl*$^{-/-}$ mouse line [79, 80]. NRL, a rod-specific transcription factor, is essential for rod differentiation [81]. The *Nrl*$^{-/-}$ mice develop a rodless and S-cone-enriched retina. These mice show no rod function but enhanced cone function [81, 82]. Using the *Nrl*$^{-/-}$ retinas, we have shown abundant expression of the cone CNG channel, and have demonstrated that CNGA3 and CNGB3 interact *in vivo* and that the cone CNG channel is a heterotetrameric complex [83]. Similar to their respective single knockout mice, *Cnga3*$^{-/-}$/*Nrl*$^{-/-}$ and *Cngb3*$^{-/-}$/*Nrl*$^{-/-}$ mice show cone dysfunction and cone loss due to apoptosis [79, 80]. In addition to mouse models, canine models of CNGB3 deficiency/mutations have been used to examine CNG channel-associated cone defects and in therapeutic interventions [51, 61, 67, 68].

Mechanisms of Cone Degeneration Due to CNG Channel Deficiency

As cones are the minority photoreceptor population in mammalian retina, examining cone dysfunction represents a major challenge. The double knockout

Cnga3$^{-/-}$/Nrl$^{-/-}$ and *Cngb3$^{-/-}$/Nrl$^{-/-}$* mice serve as excellent platform to study the modes of cone defects in CNG channel deficiency. Much of our understanding of the cellular alterations in cones lacking functional CNG channels was obtained from studies using these mice.

Endoplasmic Reticulum Stress-Associated Cone Death

CNG channel-deficient mice display early-onset apoptotic cone death [70, 79]. Using the double mutant mice, we showed that apoptotic cone death is associated with endoplasmic reticulum (ER) stress [79]. These results were further corroborated by the identification of significant upregulation of the genes involved in eIF2/ER stress in the double mutant retinas [80]. ER stress also manifested as impaired opsin trafficking/outer segment localization in *Cnga3$^{-/-}$* and *Cngb3$^{-/-}$* mice [64, 70, 73]. In the retinas of these mice, opsin co-localized with Grp78/Bip in the inner segments, supporting the accumulation of cone opsin in the ER [79]. It is worth mentioning that the increases in the ER stress marker proteins were more prominent in *Cnga3$^{-/-}$/Nrl$^{-/-}$* retinas than in *Cngb3$^{-/-}$/Nrl$^{-/-}$* retinas, suggesting relatively severe ER stress in the *Cnga3$^{-/-}$/Nrl$^{-/-}$* retinas [79, 80]. CNGA3 deficiency causes a loss of cone function while CNGB3 absence leads to reduced cone function. Using the ER chemical chaperone tauroursodeoxycholic acid (TUDCA), we further demonstrated the contribution of ER stress to cone death. Treatment with TUDCA significantly reduced ER stress and cone apoptosis, and improved cone survival in *Cnga3$^{-/-}$/Nrl$^{-/-}$* mice [80]. Indeed, ER stress has been previously documented in rod degenerations, including those caused by mutations in rhodopsin [84 - 87] and PDE6 [88 - 90].

Persistent ER stress triggers apoptosis [91 - 94]. ER stress-mediated cone death is likely mediated by the following two pathways (1). *The Grp78/Bip-eIF2a-CHOP pathway.* It is known that ER stress [95] and alterations of Ca^{2+} flux across the ER membrane [96] induce CHOP. CNG channel-deficient retinas show increased levels of CHOP and elevations of Grp78/Bip and phospho-eIF2a [79], implying an ER stress-activated, CHOP-mediated cell death. (2). *The calpain-caspase-7/12 pathway.* Calpains are known to be activated in ER stress and mediate caspase-12 processing [91, 97]. The processed forms translocate to the nucleus to induce apoptosis [98]. See Fig. (1) for details. *Cnga3$^{-/-}$/Nrl$^{-/-}$* and *Cngb3$^{-/-}$/Nrl$^{-/-}$* retinas show increased expression of calpains, enhanced caspase-12 processing, and nuclear localization of the processed forms [79], supporting that caspase-12 might act as an executioner caspase. Calpains cleave caspase-7 [99], generating highly active fragments of caspase-7, which cleave caspase-12 [99]. The full-length caspase-7 was universally detected, while the processed forms were found mainly in the *Cnga3$^{-/-}$/Nrl$^{-/-}$* and *Cngb3$^{-/-}$/Nrl$^{-/-}$* retinas [79]. Hence, activated caspase-7 might also play a role in cone death. Although the exact mechanism(s) of ER stress remain to be determined, an altered cellular calcium homeostasis might be partly responsible. As a Ca^{2+} storage organelle, the ER is sensitive to cellular Ca^{2+} levels. The CNG channel is the only source for Ca^{2+} influx in the outer segments [6]. In the absence of functional CNG channel the inward Ca^{2+} currents are abolished, which potentially results in the lowering of cellular Ca^{2+} levels.

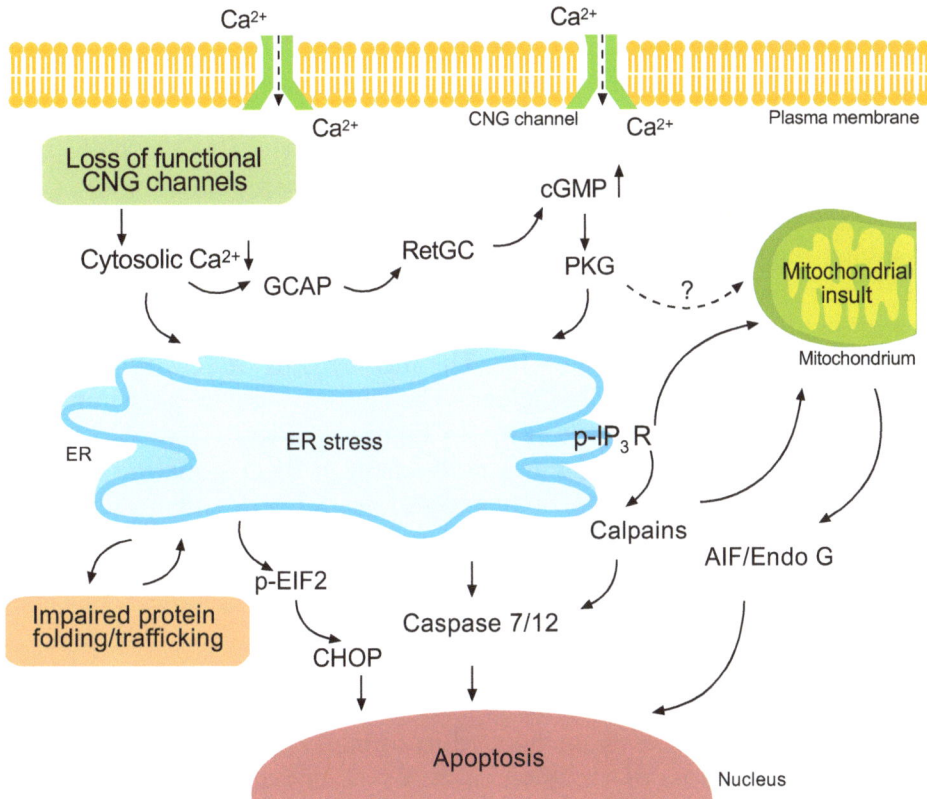

Fig. (1). Cellular mechanisms of apoptotic cone death. Loss of functional CNG channel leads to impaired cytosolic calcium homeostasis and elevation of cGMP/PKG signaling, which elicit UPR and ER stress. Such ER stress triggers apoptotic death through activation of CHOP, caspase-7/12 and AIF/Endo G pathways. Protein folding and trafficking is impaired, which further worsens the ER stress situations. The cGMP/PKG signaling might induce mitochondrial insult through unknown mechanism(s).

cGMP Accumulation and Cone Death in CNG Channel Deficiency

CNG channel-deficient retinas show a remarkable elevation of the cellular cGMP level [66, 78, 100], reflecting reduced cytosolic Ca^{2+} levels. Retinal cGMP level in *Cnga3⁻/⁻/Nrl⁻/⁻* mice increased at postnatal day 8 (P8), with maximum levels at P10-15 with an approximately 50-fold increase as compared to age-matched controls, remained higher around P30-60, and reduced to near control levels at P90 [78]. The cGMP elevation pattern correlated with apoptotic cone death, which peaked around P15-20 [70, 79]. The elevation of the cyclic monophosphate was only for cGMP but not for cAMP [78] though cAMP was elevated in several retinal degeneration models [101, 102]. The contribution of cGMP accumulation to cone death is demonstrated by work with *Cnga3$^{-/-}$/Gucy2e$^{-/-}$* mice lacking retinal guanylate cyclase-1 (retGC1). Cone density analysis using cone-specific markers showed significantly better cone survival in *Cnga3$^{-/-}$/Gucy2e$^{-/-}$* mice. M-opsin and S-opsin labeling increased by about 1-2 fold in *Cnga3$^{-/-}$/Gucy2e$^{-/-}$* mice, compared with that in age-matched *Cnga3$^{-/-}$* mice [78]. The *Cnga3$^{-/-}$/Gucy2e$^{-/-}$* mice also exhibited increased expression of M-opsin, S-opsin, GNAT2, and cone arrestin [78]. The improved cone survival in *Cnga3$^{-/-}$/Gucy2e$^{-/-}$* mice was detected from 1-9 months of age [78]. However, the cone density in the *Cnga3$^{-/-}$/Gucy2e$^{-/-}$* mice was similar to that of the *Gucy2e$^{-/-}$* mice [78]. Indeed, accumulation of cGMP has been associated with photoreceptor cytotoxicity in PDE6 deficiency [103, 104] or in guanylate cyclase activating protein (GCAP) mutations that cause activation of retGC in the dark [105]. The contribution of cGMP accumulation to cone death indicates that the cxytotoxic effects of cGMP accumulation in photoreceptors are independent of CNG channel activity. The mechanisms of cGMP accumulation-dependent cell death are still unclear. The activity and expression levels of cGMP-dependent protein kinase (protein kinase G, PKG) were elevated in the *Cnga3$^{-/-}$/Nrl$^{-/-}$* retinas, suggesting an involvement of PKG signaling in cell death [78]. cGMP/PKG signaling contributes to rod death in *rd1* mice. Treatment with PKG inhibitor resulted in photoreceptor protection in *rd1* mice [106].

Accumulation of cGMP in CNG channel-deficient retina is likely a consequence of overproduction. As PDE6 enzyme activity was not reduced [78], it suggested that the increased cGMP levels are not caused by reduced degradation. Moreover, the GC activity was not increased and the expression of the cone Na$^+$/Ca^{2+}-K$^+$ exchanger NCKX2 [83], was unchanged in *Cnga3$^{-/-}$/Nrl$^{-/-}$* retinas [78]. Based on the functional features of photoreceptor CNG channels and the regulatory mechanisms of cGMP production in photoreceptors, the elevation of cGMP is most likely a result of reduced cytosolic Ca^{2+} levels. In photoreceptors, production of cGMP is tightly regulated by intracellular Ca^{2+} *via* the GCAP-retGC axis [107 - 111]. Low Ca^{2+} concentration stimulates retGC *via* GCAP. The potentially lowered cellular Ca^{2+} level in the CNG channel-deficient cones is supported by increased phosphorylation of IP$_3$R and elevated expression of Bcl-2 [79]. Bcl-2 modulates Ca^{2+} release from ER storage to compensate for the low cytosolic Ca^{2+} levels [112].

Mitochondrial Insult in CNG Channel Deficiency

ER stress and calpain activation insults mitochondria, manifested as increased mitochondrial membrane permeability and release of apoptosis inducing factor (AIF) [88, 113, 114]. AIF is known to trigger chromatin condensation and DNA degradation [115]. When the mitochondria are damaged, AIF moves from the membrane to the cytosol and initiates caspase-independent cell death [114]. The released AIF can also translocate into the nucleus and induce DNA fragmentation [115]. Several animal models, including the *rd1* mice [88, 113], RCS rats [116], and *Uchl3*[-/-] mice [117], exhibit activation of calpains and AIF in the retina. We found increased AIF levels in the nuclear fractions of CNG channel-deficient retinas [79]. Elevated expression of mitochondrial apoptotic proteins in *Cnga3*[-/-]*/Nrl*[-/-] and *Cngb3*[-/-]*/Nrl*[-/-] retinas suggests a potential mitochondrial insult in CNG channel deficiency. The increased AIF and elevated calpains suggest activated calpain-AIF pathway that involved both ER and mitochondria functions. Endonuclease G (Endo G) is an endonuclease that is localized in mitochondria, and acts as an apoptotic DNase when released from mitochondria [118]. We found significantly elevated Endo G in *Cnga3*[-/-]*/Nrl*[-/-] and *Cngb3*[-/-]*/Nrl*[-/-] retinas [79], suggesting mitochondria-related cell death regulation in CNG channel deficiency.

CONCLUDING REMARKS

Lack of functional CNG channel triggers degeneration and death of cone photoreceptors by induction of several cellular events and multiple mechanisms (Fig. **1**). Cones lacking functional CNG channels undergo early onset, ER-stres--associated apoptosis, which is primarily mediated by the Grp78/Bip-eIF2--CHOP pathway. ER stress is likely a result of the perturbation of cellular calcium and increased cGMP/PKG signaling. Accumulation of cellular cGMP is a result of the reduced cellular Ca^{2+} level that is directly caused by loss of the functional channel. The target deletion study demonstrates that cGMP accumulation partly contributes to cone death. ER stress may also affect mitochondrial function *via* calpains and IP_3R, and lead to AIF/Endo G activation. Future efforts should be directed toward understanding how ER stress takes place in CNG channel deficiency and whether non-apoptotic cell death is involved.

CONFLICT OF INTEREST

The author (editor) declares no conflict of interest, financial or otherwise.

ACKNOWLEDGEMENTS

This work was supported by grants from the National Eye Institute (P30EY021725 and R01EY019490), the Oklahoma Center for the Advancement of Science and Technology (OCAST), and the Deutsche Forschungsgemeinschaft (DFG). We thank Drs. Anand Swaroop and Wolfgang Baehr for providing the *Nrl*[-/-] and *Gucy2e*[-/-] mouse lines.

REFERENCES

[1]   Kaupp UB, Niidome T, Tanabe T, *et al.* Primary structure and functional expression from complementary DNA of the rod photoreceptor cyclic GMP-gated channel. Nature 1989; 342(6251): 762-6.
[http://dx.doi.org/10.1038/342762a0] [PMID: 2481236]

[2]   Hirano AA, Hack I, Wässle H, Duvoisin RM. Cloning and immunocytochemical localization of a cyclic nucleotide-gated channel alpha-subunit to all cone photoreceptors in the mouse retina. J Comp Neurol 2000; 421(1): 80-94.
[http://dx.doi.org/10.1002/(SICI)1096-9861(20000522)421:1<80::AID-CNE5>3.0.CO;2-O] [PMID: 10813773]

[3]   Bönigk W, Altenhofen W, Müller F, *et al.* Rod and cone photoreceptor cells express distinct genes for cGMP-gated channels. Neuron 1993; 10(5): 865-77.
[http://dx.doi.org/10.1016/0896-6273(93)90202-3] [PMID: 7684234]

[4]   Biel M, Zong X, Ludwig A, Sautter A, Hofmann F. Molecular cloning and expression of the Modulatory subunit of the cyclic nucleotide-gated cation channel. J Biol Chem 1996; 271(11): 6349-55.
[http://dx.doi.org/10.1074/jbc.271.11.6349] [PMID: 8626431]

[5]   Pugh EN Jr aLT. Handbook of Biological Physics. edited by Stavenga DG DW, and Pugh EN, Jr., editor. Amsterdam: Elsevier/North-Holland 2000; 183.

[6]   Kaupp UB, Seifert R. Cyclic nucleotide-gated ion channels. Physiol Rev 2002; 82(3): 769-824.
[http://dx.doi.org/10.1152/physrev.00008.2002] [PMID: 12087135]

[7]   Biel M, Michalakis S. Cyclic nucleotide-gated channels. Handb Exp Pharmacol 2009; (191): 111-36.
[http://dx.doi.org/10.1007/978-3-540-68964-5_7] [PMID: 19089328]

[8]   Biel M. Cyclic nucleotide-regulated cation channels. J Biol Chem 2009; 284(14): 9017-21.
[http://dx.doi.org/10.1074/jbc.R800075200] [PMID: 19054768]

[9]   Gerstner A, Zong X, Hofmann F, Biel M. Molecular cloning and functional characterization of a new modulatory cyclic nucleotide-gated channel subunit from mouse retina. J Neurosci 2000; 20(4): 1324-32.
[PMID: 10662822]

[10]   Zagotta WN, Siegelbaum SA. Structure and function of cyclic nucleotide-gated channels. Annu Rev Neurosci 1996; 19: 235-63.
[http://dx.doi.org/10.1146/annurev.ne.19.030196.001315] [PMID: 8833443]

[11]   Okada A, Ueyama H, Toyoda F, *et al.* Functional role of hCngb3 in regulation of human cone cng channel: effect of rod monochromacy-associated mutations in hCNGB3 on channel function. Invest Ophthalmol Vis Sci 2004; 45(7): 2324-32.
[http://dx.doi.org/10.1167/iovs.03-1094] [PMID: 15223812]

[12]   Dryja TP, Finn JT, Peng YW, McGee TL, Berson EL, Yau KW. Mutations in the gene encoding the alpha subunit of the rod cGMP-gated channel in autosomal recessive retinitis pigmentosa. Proc Natl Acad Sci USA 1995; 92(22): 10177-81.
[http://dx.doi.org/10.1073/pnas.92.22.10177] [PMID: 7479749]

[13]   Trudeau MC, Zagotta WN. An intersubunit interaction regulates trafficking of rod cyclic nucleotide-gated channels and is disrupted in an inherited form of blindness. Neuron 2002; 34(2): 197-207.
[http://dx.doi.org/10.1016/S0896-6273(02)00647-5] [PMID: 11970862]

[14]   Bareil C, Hamel CP, Delague V, Arnaud B, Demaille J, Claustres M. Segregation of a mutation in CNGB1 encoding the beta-subunit of the rod cGMP-gated channel in a family with autosomal recessive retinitis pigmentosa. Hum Genet 2001; 108(4): 328-34.
[http://dx.doi.org/10.1007/s004390100496] [PMID: 11379879]

[15]   Kohl S, Marx T, Giddings I, *et al*. Total colourblindness is caused by mutations in the gene encoding the alpha-subunit of the cone photoreceptor cGMP-gated cation channel. Nat Genet 1998; 19(3): 257-9.
[http://dx.doi.org/10.1038/935] [PMID: 9662398]

[16]   Wissinger B, Gamer D, Jägle H, *et al*. CNGA3 mutations in hereditary cone photoreceptor disorders. Am J Hum Genet 2001; 69(4): 722-37.
[http://dx.doi.org/10.1086/323613] [PMID: 11536077]

[17]   Nishiguchi KM, Sandberg MA, Gorji N, Berson EL, Dryja TP. Cone cGMP-gated channel mutations and clinical findings in patients with achromatopsia, macular degeneration, and other hereditary cone diseases. Hum Mutat 2005; 25(3): 248-58.
[http://dx.doi.org/10.1002/humu.20142] [PMID: 15712225]

[18]   Kohl S, Baumann B, Broghammer M, *et al*. Mutations in the CNGB3 gene encoding the beta-subunit of the cone photoreceptor cGMP-gated channel are responsible for achromatopsia (ACHM3) linked to chromosome 8q21. Hum Mol Genet 2000; 9(14): 2107-16.
[http://dx.doi.org/10.1093/hmg/9.14.2107] [PMID: 10958649]

[19]   Wawrocka A, Kohl S, Baumann B, *et al*. Five novel CNGB3 gene mutations in Polish patients with achromatopsia. Mol Vis 2014; 20: 1732-9.
[PMID: 25558176]

[20]   Wang X, Wang H, Cao M, *et al*. Whole-exome sequencing identifies ALMS1, IQCB1, CNGA3, and MYO7A mutations in patients with Leber congenital amaurosis. Hum Mutat 2011; 32(12): 1450-9.
[http://dx.doi.org/10.1002/humu.21587] [PMID: 21901789]

[21]   Kohl S, Varsanyi B, Antunes GA, *et al*. CNGB3 mutations account for 50% of all cases with autosomal recessive achromatopsia. Eur J Hum Genet 2005; 13(3): 302-8.
[http://dx.doi.org/10.1038/sj.ejhg.5201269] [PMID: 15657609]

[22]   Li S, Huang L, Xiao X, Jia X, Guo X, Zhang Q. Identification of CNGA3 mutations in 46 families: common cause of achromatopsia and cone-rod dystrophies in Chinese patients. JAMA Ophthalmol 2014; 132(9): 1076-83.
[http://dx.doi.org/10.1001/jamaophthalmol.2014.1032] [PMID: 24903488]

[23]   Liang X, Dong F, Li H, Li H, Yang L, Sui R. Novel CNGA3 mutations in Chinese patients with achromatopsia. Br J Ophthalmol 2015; 99(4): 571-6.
[http://dx.doi.org/10.1136/bjophthalmol-2014-305432] [PMID: 25637600]

[24]   Zelinger L, Cideciyan AV, Kohl S, *et al*. Genetics and Disease Expression in the CNGA3 Form of Achromatopsia: Steps on the Path to Gene Therapy. Ophthalmology 2015; 122(5): 997-1007.
[http://dx.doi.org/10.1016/j.ophtha.2014.11.025] [PMID: 25616768]

[25]   Doucette L, Green J, Black C, *et al*. Molecular genetics of achromatopsia in Newfoundland reveal genetic heterogeneity, founder effects and the first cases of Jalili syndrome in North America. Ophthalmic Genet 2013; 34(3): 119-29.
[http://dx.doi.org/10.3109/13816810.2013.763993] [PMID: 23362848]

[26]   Schön C, Biel M, Michalakis S. Gene replacement therapy for retinal CNG channelopathies. Mol Genet Genomics 2013; 288(10): 459-67.
[http://dx.doi.org/10.1007/s00438-013-0766-4] [PMID: 23861024]

[27]   Ben Simon GJ, Abraham FA, Melamed S. Pingelapese achromatopsia: correlation between paradoxical pupillary response and clinical features. Br J Ophthalmol 2004; 88(2): 223-5.
[http://dx.doi.org/10.1136/bjo.2003.027284] [PMID: 14736779]

[28]   Andréasson S, Tornqvist K. Electroretinograms in patients with achromatopsia. Acta Ophthalmol (Copenh) 1991; 69(6): 711-6.
[http://dx.doi.org/10.1111/j.1755-3768.1991.tb02048.x] [PMID: 1789084]

[29]   Khan NW, Wissinger B, Kohl S, Sieving PA. CNGB3 achromatopsia with progressive loss of residual

cone function and impaired rod-mediated function. Invest Ophthalmol Vis Sci 2007; 48(8): 3864-71.
[http://dx.doi.org/10.1167/iovs.06-1521] [PMID: 17652762]

[30]   Varsányi B, Somfai GM, Lesch B, Vámos R, Farkas A. Optical coherence tomography of the macula in congenital achromatopsia. Invest Ophthalmol Vis Sci 2007; 48(5): 2249-53.
[http://dx.doi.org/10.1167/iovs.06-1173] [PMID: 17460287]

[31]   Thiadens AA, Somervuo V, van den Born LI, *et al.* Progressive loss of cones in achromatopsia: an imaging study using spectral-domain optical coherence tomography. Invest Ophthalmol Vis Sci 2010; 51(11): 5952-7.
[http://dx.doi.org/10.1167/iovs.10-5680] [PMID: 20574029]

[32]   Genead MA, Fishman GA, Rha J, *et al.* Photoreceptor structure and function in patients with congenital achromatopsia. Invest Ophthalmol Vis Sci 2011; 52(10): 7298-308.
[http://dx.doi.org/10.1167/iovs.11-7762] [PMID: 21778272]

[33]   Yang P, Michaels KV, Courtney RJ, *et al.* Retinal morphology of patients with achromatopsia during early childhood: implications for gene therapy. JAMA Ophthalmol 2014; 132(7): 823-31.
[http://dx.doi.org/10.1001/jamaophthalmol.2014.685] [PMID: 24676353]

[34]   McClintock M, Peden MC, Kay CN. Spectral domain optical coherence tomography findings in CNGB3-associated achromatopsia and therapeutic implications. Adv Exp Med Biol 2014; 801: 551-7.
[http://dx.doi.org/10.1007/978-1-4614-3209-8_70] [PMID: 24664743]

[35]   Greenberg JP, Sherman J, Zweifel SA, *et al.* Spectral-domain optical coherence tomography staging and autofluorescence imaging in achromatopsia. JAMA Ophthalmol 2014; 132(4): 437-45.
[http://dx.doi.org/10.1001/jamaophthalmol.2013.7987] [PMID: 24504161]

[36]   Fahim AT, Khan NW, Zahid S, Schachar IH, Branham K, Kohl S, *et al.* Diagnostic fundus autofluorescence patterns in achromatopsia. Am J Ophthalmol 2013; 156(6): 1211-9.
[http://dx.doi.org/10.1016/j.ajo.2013.06.033]

[37]   Thomas MG, McLean RJ, Kohl S, Sheth V, Gottlob I. Early signs of longitudinal progressive cone photoreceptor degeneration in achromatopsia. Br J Ophthalmol 2012; 96(9): 1232-6.
[http://dx.doi.org/10.1136/bjophthalmol-2012-301737] [PMID: 22790432]

[38]   Dubis AM, Cooper RF, Aboshiha J, *et al.* Genotype-dependent variability in residual cone structure in achromatopsia: toward developing metrics for assessing cone health. Invest Ophthalmol Vis Sci 2014; 55(11): 7303-11.
[http://dx.doi.org/10.1167/iovs.14-14225] [PMID: 25277229]

[39]   Carroll J, Choi SS, Williams DR. *In vivo* imaging of the photoreceptor mosaic of a rod monochromat. Vision Res 2008; 48(26): 2564-8.
[http://dx.doi.org/10.1016/j.visres.2008.04.006] [PMID: 18499214]

[40]   Sundin OH, Yang JM, Li Y, *et al.* Genetic basis of total colourblindness among the Pingelapese islanders. Nat Genet 2000; 25(3): 289-93.
[http://dx.doi.org/10.1038/77162] [PMID: 10888875]

[41]   Wiszniewski W, Lewis RA, Lupski JR. Achromatopsia: the CNGB3 p.T383fsX mutation results from a founder effect and is responsible for the visual phenotype in the original report of uniparental disomy 14. Hum Genet 2007; 121(3-4): 433-9.
[http://dx.doi.org/10.1007/s00439-006-0314-y] [PMID: 17265047]

[42]   Saqib MA, Awan BM, Sarfraz M, Khan MN, Rashid S, Ansar M. Genetic analysis of four Pakistani families with achromatopsia and a novel S4 motif mutation of CNGA3. Jpn J Ophthalmol 2011; 55(6): 676-80.
[http://dx.doi.org/10.1007/s10384-011-0070-y] [PMID: 21912902]

[43]   Lam K, Guo H, Wilson GA, Kohl S, Wong F. Identification of variants in CNGA3 as cause for achromatopsia by exome sequencing of a single patient. Arch Ophthalmol 2011; 129(9): 1212-7.
[http://dx.doi.org/10.1001/archophthalmol.2011.254] [PMID: 21911670]

[44]   Zelinger L, Greenberg A, Kohl S, Banin E, Sharon D. An ancient autosomal haplotype bearing a rare achromatopsia-causing founder mutation is shared among Arab Muslims and Oriental Jews. Hum Genet 2010; 128(3): 261-7.
[http://dx.doi.org/10.1007/s00439-010-0846-z] [PMID: 20549516]

[45]   Azam M, Collin RW, Shah ST, *et al.* Novel CNGA3 and CNGB3 mutations in two Pakistani families with achromatopsia. Mol Vis 2010; 16: 774-81.
[PMID: 20454696]

[46]   Ahuja Y, Kohl S, Traboulsi EI. CNGA3 mutations in two United Arab Emirates families with achromatopsia. Mol Vis 2008; 14: 1293-7.
[PMID: 18636117]

[47]   Patel KA, Bartoli KM, Fandino RA, *et al.* Transmembrane S1 mutations in CNGA3 from achromatopsia 2 patients cause loss of function and impaired cellular trafficking of the cone CNG channel. Invest Ophthalmol Vis Sci 2005; 46(7): 2282-90.
[http://dx.doi.org/10.1167/iovs.05-0179] [PMID: 15980212]

[48]   Faillace MP, Bernabeu RO, Korenbrot JI. Cellular processing of cone photoreceptor cyclic GMP-gated ion channels: a role for the S4 structural motif. J Biol Chem 2004; 279(21): 22643-53.
[http://dx.doi.org/10.1074/jbc.M400035200] [PMID: 15024024]

[49]   Liu C, Varnum MD. Functional consequences of progressive cone dystrophy-associated mutations in the human cone photoreceptor cyclic nucleotide-gated channel CNGA3 subunit. Am J Physiol Cell Physiol 2005; 289(1): C187-98.
[http://dx.doi.org/10.1152/ajpcell.00490.2004] [PMID: 15743887]

[50]   Muraki-Oda S, Toyoda F, Okada A, *et al.* Functional analysis of rod monochromacy-associated missense mutations in the CNGA3 subunit of the cone photoreceptor cGMP-gated channel. Biochem Biophys Res Commun 2007; 362(1): 88-93.
[http://dx.doi.org/10.1016/j.bbrc.2007.07.152] [PMID: 17693388]

[51]   Tanaka N, Delemotte L, Klein ML, Komáromy AM, Tanaka JC. A cyclic nucleotide-gated channel mutation associated with canine daylight blindness provides insight into a role for the S2 segment tri-Asp motif in channel biogenesis. PLoS One 2014; 9(2): e88768.
[http://dx.doi.org/10.1371/journal.pone.0088768] [PMID: 24586388]

[52]   Koeppen K, Reuter P, Ladewig T, *et al.* Dissecting the pathogenic mechanisms of mutations in the pore region of the human cone photoreceptor cyclic nucleotide-gated channel. Hum Mutat 2010; 31(7): 830-9.
[http://dx.doi.org/10.1002/humu.21283] [PMID: 20506298]

[53]   Koeppen K, Reuter P, Kohl S, Baumann B, Ladewig T, Wissinger B. Functional analysis of human CNGA3 mutations associated with colour blindness suggests impaired surface expression of channel mutants A3(R427C) and A3(R563C). Eur J Neurosci 2008; 27(9): 2391-401.
[http://dx.doi.org/10.1111/j.1460-9568.2008.06195.x] [PMID: 18445228]

[54]   Reuter P, Koeppen K, Ladewig T, Kohl S, Baumann B, Wissinger B. Mutations in CNGA3 impair trafficking or function of cone cyclic nucleotide-gated channels, resulting in achromatopsia. Hum Mutat 2008; 29(10): 1228-36.
[http://dx.doi.org/10.1002/humu.20790] [PMID: 18521937]

[55]   Tränkner D, Jägle H, Kohl S, *et al.* Molecular basis of an inherited form of incomplete achromatopsia. J Neurosci 2004; 24(1): 138-47.
[http://dx.doi.org/10.1523/JNEUROSCI.3883-03.2004] [PMID: 14715947]

[56]   Ding XQ, Fitzgerald JB, Quiambao AB, Harry CS, Malykhina AP. Molecular pathogenesis of achromatopsia associated with mutations in the cone cyclic nucleotide-gated channel CNGA3 subunit. Adv Exp Med Biol 2010; 664: 245-53.
[http://dx.doi.org/10.1007/978-1-4419-1399-9_28] [PMID: 20238023]

[57]   Matveev AV, Fitzgerald JB, Xu J, Malykhina AP, Rodgers KK, Ding XQ. The disease-causing mutations in the carboxyl terminus of the cone cyclic nucleotide-gated channel CNGA3 subunit alter the local secondary structure and interfere with the channel active conformational change. Biochemistry 2010; 49(8): 1628-39.
[http://dx.doi.org/10.1021/bi901960u] [PMID: 20088482]

[58]   Johnson S, Michaelides M, Aligianis IA, *et al.* Achromatopsia caused by novel mutations in both CNGA3 and CNGB3. J Med Genet 2004; 41(2): e20.
[http://dx.doi.org/10.1136/jmg.2003.011437] [PMID: 14757870]

[59]   Thiadens AA, Slingerland NW, Roosing S, van Schooneveld MJ, van Lith-Verhoeven JJ, van Moll-Ramirez N, *et al.* Genetic etiology and clinical consequences of complete and incomplete achromatopsia. Ophthalmology 2009; 116(10): 1984-9.
[http://dx.doi.org/10.1016/j.ophtha.2009.03.053]

[60]   Reicher S, Seroussi E, Gootwine E. A mutation in gene CNGA3 is associated with day blindness in sheep. Genomics 2010; 95(2): 101-4.
[http://dx.doi.org/10.1016/j.ygeno.2009.10.003] [PMID: 19874885]

[61]   Sidjanin DJ, Lowe JK, McElwee JL, *et al.* Canine CNGB3 mutations establish cone degeneration as orthologous to the human achromatopsia locus ACHM3. Hum Mol Genet 2002; 11(16): 1823-33.
[http://dx.doi.org/10.1093/hmg/11.16.1823] [PMID: 12140185]

[62]   Seddon JM, Hampson EC, Smith RI, Hughes IP. Genetic heterogeneity of day blindness in Alaskan Malamutes. Anim Genet 2006; 37(4): 407-10.
[http://dx.doi.org/10.1111/j.1365-2052.2006.01484.x] [PMID: 16879359]

[63]   Yeh CY, Goldstein O, Kukekova AV, *et al.* Genomic deletion of CNGB3 is identical by descent in multiple canine breeds and causes achromatopsia. BMC Genet 2013; 14: 27.
[http://dx.doi.org/10.1186/1471-2156-14-27] [PMID: 23601474]

[64]   Carvalho LS, Xu J, Pearson RA, *et al.* Long-term and age-dependent restoration of visual function in a mouse model of CNGB3-associated achromatopsia following gene therapy. Hum Mol Genet 2011; 20(16): 3161-75.
[http://dx.doi.org/10.1093/hmg/ddr218] [PMID: 21576125]

[65]   Pang JJ, Deng WT, Dai X, *et al.* AAV-mediated cone rescue in a naturally occurring mouse model of CNGA3-achromatopsia. PLoS One 2012; 7(4): e35250.
[http://dx.doi.org/10.1371/journal.pone.0035250] [PMID: 22509403]

[66]   Michalakis S, Mühlfriedel R, Tanimoto N, *et al.* Restoration of cone vision in the CNGA3-/- mouse model of congenital complete lack of cone photoreceptor function. Mol Ther 2010; 18(12): 2057-63.
[http://dx.doi.org/10.1038/mt.2010.149] [PMID: 20628362]

[67]   Komáromy AM, Alexander JJ, Rowlan JS, *et al.* Gene therapy rescues cone function in congenital achromatopsia. Hum Mol Genet 2010; 19(13): 2581-93.
[http://dx.doi.org/10.1093/hmg/ddq136] [PMID: 20378608]

[68]   Komáromy AM, Rowlan JS, Corr AT, *et al.* Transient photoreceptor deconstruction by CNTF enhances rAAV-mediated cone functional rescue in late stage CNGB3-achromatopsia. Mol Ther 2013; 21(6): 1131-41.
[http://dx.doi.org/10.1038/mt.2013.50] [PMID: 23568263]

[69]   Zein WM, Jeffrey BG, Wiley HE, *et al.* CNGB3-achromatopsia clinical trial with CNTF: diminished rod pathway responses with no evidence of improvement in cone function. Invest Ophthalmol Vis Sci 2014; 55(10): 6301-8.
[http://dx.doi.org/10.1167/iovs.14-14860] [PMID: 25205868]

[70]   Michalakis S, Geiger H, Haverkamp S, Hofmann F, Gerstner A, Biel M. Impaired opsin targeting and cone photoreceptor migration in the retina of mice lacking the cyclic nucleotide-gated channel CNGA3. Invest Ophthalmol Vis Sci 2005; 46(4): 1516-24.

[http://dx.doi.org/10.1167/iovs.04-1503] [PMID: 15790924]

[71]   Biel M, Seeliger M, Pfeifer A, *et al.* Selective loss of cone function in mice lacking the cyclic nucleotide-gated channel CNG3. Proc Natl Acad Sci USA 1999; 96(13): 7553-7.
[http://dx.doi.org/10.1073/pnas.96.13.7553] [PMID: 10377453]

[72]   Ding XQ, Harry CS, Umino Y, Matveev AV, Fliesler SJ, Barlow RB. Impaired cone function and cone degeneration resulting from CNGB3 deficiency: down-regulation of CNGA3 biosynthesis as a potential mechanism. Hum Mol Genet 2009; 18(24): 4770-80.
[http://dx.doi.org/10.1093/hmg/ddp440] [PMID: 19767295]

[73]   Xu J, Morris L, Fliesler SJ, Sherry DM, Ding XQ. Early-onset, slow progression of cone photoreceptor dysfunction and degeneration in CNG channel subunit CNGB3 deficiency. Invest Ophthalmol Vis Sci 2011; 52(6): 3557-66.
[http://dx.doi.org/10.1167/iovs.10-6358] [PMID: 21273547]

[74]   Xu J, Morris LM, Michalakis S, *et al.* CNGA3 deficiency affects cone synaptic terminal structure and function and leads to secondary rod dysfunction and degeneration. Invest Ophthalmol Vis Sci 2012; 53(3): 1117-29.
[http://dx.doi.org/10.1167/iovs.11-8168] [PMID: 22247469]

[75]   Haverkamp S, Michalakis S, Claes E, *et al.* Synaptic plasticity in CNGA3(-/-) mice: cone bipolar cells react on the missing cone input and form ectopic synapses with rods. J Neurosci 2006; 26(19): 5248-55.
[http://dx.doi.org/10.1523/JNEUROSCI.4483-05.2006] [PMID: 16687517]

[76]   Michalakis S, Kleppisch T, Polta SA, *et al.* Altered synaptic plasticity and behavioral abnormalities in CNGA3-deficient mice. Genes Brain Behav 2011; 10(2): 137-48.
[http://dx.doi.org/10.1111/j.1601-183X.2010.00646.x] [PMID: 20846178]

[77]   Schmucker C, Seeliger M, Humphries P, Biel M, Schaeffel F. Grating acuity at different luminances in wild-type mice and in mice lacking rod or cone function. Invest Ophthalmol Vis Sci 2005; 46(1): 398-407.
[http://dx.doi.org/10.1167/iovs.04-0959] [PMID: 15623801]

[78]   Xu J, Morris L, Thapa A, *et al.* cGMP accumulation causes photoreceptor degeneration in CNG channel deficiency: evidence of cGMP cytotoxicity independently of enhanced CNG channel function. J Neurosci 2013; 33(37): 14939-48.
[http://dx.doi.org/10.1523/JNEUROSCI.0909-13.2013] [PMID: 24027293]

[79]   Thapa A, Morris L, Xu J, *et al.* Endoplasmic reticulum stress-associated cone photoreceptor degeneration in cyclic nucleotide-gated channel deficiency. J Biol Chem 2012; 287(22): 18018-29.
[http://dx.doi.org/10.1074/jbc.M112.342220] [PMID: 22493484]

[80]   Ma H, Thapa A, Morris LM, *et al.* Loss of cone cyclic nucleotide-gated channel leads to alterations in light response modulating system and cellular stress response pathways: a gene expression profiling study. Hum Mol Genet 2013; 22(19): 3906-19.
[http://dx.doi.org/10.1093/hmg/ddt245] [PMID: 23740940]

[81]   Mears AJ, Kondo M, Swain PK, *et al.* Nrl is required for rod photoreceptor development. Nat Genet 2001; 29(4): 447-52.
[http://dx.doi.org/10.1038/ng774] [PMID: 11694879]

[82]   Nikonov SS, Daniele LL, Zhu X, Craft CM, Swaroop A, Pugh EN Jr. Photoreceptors of Nrl -/- mice coexpress functional S- and M-cone opsins having distinct inactivation mechanisms. J Gen Physiol 2005; 125(3): 287-304.
[http://dx.doi.org/10.1085/jgp.200409208] [PMID: 15738050]

[83]   Matveev AV, Quiambao AB, Browning Fitzgerald J, Ding XQ. Native cone photoreceptor cyclic nucleotide-gated channel is a heterotetrameric complex comprising both CNGA3 and CNGB3: a study using the cone-dominant retina of Nrl-/- mice. J Neurochem 2008; 106(5): 2042-55.
[PMID: 18665891]

[84] Tam BM, Xie G, Oprian DD, Moritz OL. Mislocalized rhodopsin does not require activation to cause retinal degeneration and neurite outgrowth in Xenopus laevis. J Neurosci 2006; 26(1): 203-9.
[http://dx.doi.org/10.1523/JNEUROSCI.3849-05.2006] [PMID: 16399688]

[85] Griciuc A, Aron L, Piccoli G, Ueffing M. Clearance of Rhodopsin(P23H) aggregates requires the ERAD effector VCP. Biochim Biophys Acta 2010; 1803(3): 424-34.
[http://dx.doi.org/10.1016/j.bbamcr.2010.01.008] [PMID: 20097236]

[86] Griciuc A, Aron L, Roux MJ, Klein R, Giangrande A, Ueffing M. Inactivation of VCP/ter94 suppresses retinal pathology caused by misfolded rhodopsin in Drosophila. PLoS Genet 2010; 6(8): e1001075.
[http://dx.doi.org/10.1371/journal.pgen.1001075] [PMID: 20865169]

[87] Tam BM, Moritz OL. Characterization of rhodopsin P23H-induced retinal degeneration in a Xenopus laevis model of retinitis pigmentosa. Invest Ophthalmol Vis Sci 2006; 47(8): 3234-41.
[http://dx.doi.org/10.1167/iovs.06-0213] [PMID: 16877386]

[88] Sanges D, Comitato A, Tammaro R, Marigo V. Apoptosis in retinal degeneration involves cross-talk between apoptosis-inducing factor (AIF) and caspase-12 and is blocked by calpain inhibitors. Proc Natl Acad Sci USA 2006; 103(46): 17366-71.
[http://dx.doi.org/10.1073/pnas.0606276103] [PMID: 17088543]

[89] Yang LP, Wu LM, Guo XJ, Tso MO. Activation of endoplasmic reticulum stress in degenerating photoreceptors of the rd1 mouse. Invest Ophthalmol Vis Sci 2007; 48(11): 5191-8.
[http://dx.doi.org/10.1167/iovs.07-0512] [PMID: 17962473]

[90] Paquet-Durand F, Azadi S, Hauck SM, Ueffing M, van Veen T, Ekström P. Calpain is activated in degenerating photoreceptors in the rd1 mouse. J Neurochem 2006; 96(3): 802-14.
[http://dx.doi.org/10.1111/j.1471-4159.2005.03628.x] [PMID: 16405498]

[91] Nakagawa T, Zhu H, Morishima N, et al. Caspase-12 mediates endoplasmic-reticulum-specific apoptosis and cytotoxicity by amyloid-beta. Nature 2000; 403(6765): 98-103.
[http://dx.doi.org/10.1038/47513] [PMID: 10638761]

[92] Szegezdi E, Logue SE, Gorman AM, Samali A. Mediators of endoplasmic reticulum stress-induced apoptosis. EMBO Rep 2006; 7(9): 880-5.
[http://dx.doi.org/10.1038/sj.embor.7400779] [PMID: 16953201]

[93] Scull CM, Tabas I. Mechanisms of ER stress-induced apoptosis in atherosclerosis. Arterioscler Thromb Vasc Biol 2011; 31(12): 2792-7.
[http://dx.doi.org/10.1161/ATVBAHA.111.224881] [PMID: 22096099]

[94] Tabas I, Ron D. Integrating the mechanisms of apoptosis induced by endoplasmic reticulum stress. Nat Cell Biol 2011; 13(3): 184-90.
[http://dx.doi.org/10.1038/ncb0311-184] [PMID: 21364565]

[95] Li J, Lee B, Lee AS. Endoplasmic reticulum stress-induced apoptosis: multiple pathways and activation of p53-up-regulated modulator of apoptosis (PUMA) and NOXA by p53. J Biol Chem 2006; 281(11): 7260-70.
[http://dx.doi.org/10.1074/jbc.M509868200] [PMID: 16407291]

[96] Wang XZ, Lawson B, Brewer JW, et al. Signals from the stressed endoplasmic reticulum induce C/EBP-homologous protein (CHOP/GADD153). Mol Cell Biol 1996; 16(8): 4273-80.
[http://dx.doi.org/10.1128/MCB.16.8.4273] [PMID: 8754828]

[97] Nakagawa T, Yuan J. Cross-talk between two cysteine protease families. Activation of caspase-12 by calpain in apoptosis. J Cell Biol 2000; 150(4): 887-94.
[http://dx.doi.org/10.1083/jcb.150.4.887] [PMID: 10953012]

[98] Fujita E, Kouroku Y, Jimbo A, Isoai A, Maruyama K, Momoi T. Caspase-12 processing and fragment translocation into nuclei of tunicamycin-treated cells. Cell Death Differ 2002; 9(10): 1108-14.
[http://dx.doi.org/10.1038/sj.cdd.4401080] [PMID: 12232799]

[99]   Rao RV, Hermel E, Castro-Obregon S, *et al.* Coupling endoplasmic reticulum stress to the cell death program. Mechanism of caspase activation. J Biol Chem 2001; 276(36): 33869-74.
[http://dx.doi.org/10.1074/jbc.M102225200] [PMID: 11448953]

[100] Arango-Gonzalez B, Trifunović D, Sahaboglu A, *et al.* Identification of a common non-apoptotic cell death mechanism in hereditary retinal degeneration. PLoS One 2014; 9(11): e112142.
[http://dx.doi.org/10.1371/journal.pone.0112142] [PMID: 25392995]

[101] Lolley RN, Schmidt SY, Farber DB. Alterations in cyclic AMP metabolism associated with photoreceptor cell degeneration in the C3H mouse. J Neurochem 1974; 22(5): 701-7.
[http://dx.doi.org/10.1111/j.1471-4159.1974.tb04283.x] [PMID: 4366113]

[102] Weiss ER, Hao Y, Dickerson CD, *et al.* Altered cAMP levels in retinas from transgenic mice expressing a rhodopsin mutant. Biochem Biophys Res Commun 1995; 216(3): 755-61.
[http://dx.doi.org/10.1006/bbrc.1995.2686] [PMID: 7488190]

[103] Frasson M, Sahel JA, Fabre M, Simonutti M, Dreyfus H, Picaud S. Retinitis pigmentosa: rod photoreceptor rescue by a calcium-channel blocker in the rd mouse. Nat Med 1999; 5(10): 1183-7.
[http://dx.doi.org/10.1038/13508] [PMID: 10502823]

[104] Paquet-Durand F, Beck S, Michalakis S, *et al.* A key role for cyclic nucleotide gated (CNG) channels in cGMP-related retinitis pigmentosa. Hum Mol Genet 2011; 20(5): 941-7.
[http://dx.doi.org/10.1093/hmg/ddq539] [PMID: 21149284]

[105] Woodruff ML, Olshevskaya EV, Savchenko AB, *et al.* Constitutive excitation by Gly90Asp rhodopsin rescues rods from degeneration caused by elevated production of cGMP in the dark. J Neurosci 2007; 27(33): 8805-15.
[http://dx.doi.org/10.1523/JNEUROSCI.2751-07.2007] [PMID: 17699662]

[106] Paquet-Durand F, Hauck SM, van Veen T, Ueffing M, Ekström P. PKG activity causes photoreceptor cell death in two retinitis pigmentosa models. J Neurochem 2009; 108(3): 796-810.
[http://dx.doi.org/10.1111/j.1471-4159.2008.05822.x] [PMID: 19187097]

[107] Tucker CL, Woodcock SC, Kelsell RE, Ramamurthy V, Hunt DM, Hurley JB. Biochemical analysis of a dimerization domain mutation in RetGC-1 associated with dominant cone-rod dystrophy. Proc Natl Acad Sci USA 1999; 96(16): 9039-44.
[http://dx.doi.org/10.1073/pnas.96.16.9039] [PMID: 10430891]

[108] Peshenko IV, Olshevskaya EV, Savchenko AB, *et al.* Enzymatic properties and regulation of the native isozymes of retinal membrane guanylyl cyclase (RetGC) from mouse photoreceptors. Biochemistry 2011; 50(25): 5590-600.
[http://dx.doi.org/10.1021/bi200491b] [PMID: 21598940]

[109] Makino CL, Peshenko IV, Wen XH, Olshevskaya EV, Barrett R, Dizhoor AM. A role for GCAP2 in regulating the photoresponse. Guanylyl cyclase activation and rod electrophysiology in GUCA1B knock-out mice. J Biol Chem 2008; 283(43): 29135-43.
[http://dx.doi.org/10.1074/jbc.M804445200] [PMID: 18723510]

[110] Gross OP, Pugh EN Jr, Burns ME. cGMP in mouse rods: the spatiotemporal dynamics underlying single photon responses. Front Mol Neurosci 2015; 8: 6.
[http://dx.doi.org/10.3389/fnmol.2015.00006] [PMID: 25788876]

[111] Sharma RK. Membrane guanylate cyclase is a beautiful signal transduction machine: overview. Mol Cell Biochem 2010; 334(1-2): 3-36.
[http://dx.doi.org/10.1007/s11010-009-0336-6] [PMID: 19957201]

[112] Palmer AE, Jin C, Reed JC, Tsien RY. Bcl-2-mediated alterations in endoplasmic reticulum Ca2+ analyzed with an improved genetically encoded fluorescent sensor. Proc Natl Acad Sci USA 2004; 101(50): 17404-9.
[http://dx.doi.org/10.1073/pnas.0408030101] [PMID: 15585581]

[113] Sanges D, Marigo V. Cross-talk between two apoptotic pathways activated by endoplasmic reticulum

stress: differential contribution of caspase-12 and AIF. Apoptosis 2006; 11(9): 1629-41.
[http://dx.doi.org/10.1007/s10495-006-9006-2] [PMID: 16820963]

[114] Norberg E, Gogvadze V, Ott M, *et al.* An increase in intracellular Ca2+ is required for the activation of mitochondrial calpain to release AIF during cell death. Cell Death Differ 2008; 15(12): 1857-64.
[http://dx.doi.org/10.1038/cdd.2008.123] [PMID: 18806756]

[115] Polster BM, Basañez G, Etxebarria A, Hardwick JM, Nicholls DG. Calpain I induces cleavage and release of apoptosis-inducing factor from isolated mitochondria. J Biol Chem 2005; 280(8): 6447-54.
[http://dx.doi.org/10.1074/jbc.M413269200] [PMID: 15590628]

[116] Mizukoshi S, Nakazawa M, Sato K, Ozaki T, Metoki T, Ishiguro S. Activation of mitochondrial calpain and release of apoptosis-inducing factor from mitochondria in RCS rat retinal degeneration. Exp Eye Res 2010; 91(3): 353-61.
[http://dx.doi.org/10.1016/j.exer.2010.06.004] [PMID: 20547152]

[117] Sano Y, Furuta A, Setsuie R, *et al.* Photoreceptor cell apoptosis in the retinal degeneration of Uchl3-deficient mice. Am J Pathol 2006; 169(1): 132-41.
[http://dx.doi.org/10.2353/ajpath.2006.060085] [PMID: 16816367]

[118] Li LY, Luo X, Wang X. Endonuclease G is an apoptotic DNase when released from mitochondria. Nature 2001; 412(6842): 95-9.
[http://dx.doi.org/10.1038/35083620] [PMID: 11452314]

SUBJECT INDEX

A

Ablation 102
Achromatopsia 109, 110, 111
Adaptive optics scanning light
      ophthalmoscopy (AOSLO) 110
Adult mouse photoreceptors 7
Adult photoreceptors 76
All-trans retinol 9
Alterations 59, 61, 111, 112
   cellular 111, 112
   functional 59, 61
Amacrine cells 4, 9, 57
Andhra pradesh eye disease study (APEDS)
      55
Anterior chamber 3, 56
Anterior segment 10
Anterograde motor Kinesin-II 2
Antibodies 9, 76, 77, 83
Anti-KIF3A 76
Anti-VEGF therapy 56, 66
Apoptosis 25, 54, 58, 59, 60, 61, 62, 64, 65,
      89, 91, 109, 111, 112, 114
   neural 60, 62
Apoptosis inducing factor (AIF) 114, 115
Apoptotic molecules 59
Aqueous humor 3
Arrangement 1, 8, 39
ASH domain 43, 44, 45
Association for research in vision and
      ophthalmology (ARVO) 83
Atrophy 92
Aurora Kinase A 45, 46
Autophagy 54, 60, 63
Axoneme 17, 18, 39, 40, 43, 44, 45, 74, 76,
      77, 81, 82
Axoneme formation 74

B

Bardet-Biedl syndrome (BBS) 3, 16, 19, 22,
      24, 45
Barrier 10
   blood retinal 10

Basal bodies 1, 6, 17, 18, 19, 23, 39, 43, 44,
      74, 77, 78
Bbs genes result 23
Bbs morphants 22, 23, 24
Biogenesis 86, 87, 89, 91
Bipolar cells 4, 9, 57
Blindness, congenital retinal 46
Blood vessels 10, 56
Bona fide ciliary structure 18

C

Ca^{2+}-binding protein 76, 78
Calpains 112, 115
Calyceal processes 18, 19
Cataracts 43, 46
Cause rhodopsin mistrafficking, double-
      knockout mice 81
Cell loss 91, 94
Cells 4, 9, 40, 56, 57, 59, 63, 77
   ciliated 40
   horizontal 4, 9, 57, 77
   neuronal 56
   positive 59, 63
Cell types 3, 5, 8, 9, 40, 41, 91, 92
   inner retinal 9
   mouse retinal 9
Cellular Ca^{2+} levels 113
Cellular mechanism of neurodegeneration in
      diabetic retinopathy 64
Central nervous system (CNS) 54, 62, 66
Centrin-2 78, 79
Centrioles 76, 77, 78
CGMP 8, 104, 105, 109, 114
CGMP Accumulation 113, 114, 115
CGMP concentration 8, 9
CGMP/PKG signaling 113, 114
CGMP production 110, 114
Choriocapillaris 60, 92
Choriocapillaris atrophy 86
Choroidal 10
Chromophore 8, 9
Cilia 1, 2, 3, 9, 10, 16, 17, 18, 19, 21, 23, 25,
      27, 39, 44, 45, 76, 78, 82
   bronchial 3

www.ingramcontent.com/pod-product-compliance
Lightning Source LLC
Chambersburg PA
CBHW041729210326
41598CB00008B/820